Young Skin for Life

Your Guide to Smoother, Clearer, More Beautiful Skin— At Any Age

By Julie Davis
and the Editors of *PREVENTION* Magazine

Medical Adviser: Albert M. Kligman, M.D., Ph.D., Professor of Dermatology, University of Pennsylvania School of Medicine

Rodale Press, Inc.
Emmaus, Pennsylvania

Notice

This book is intended as a reference volume only, not as a medical manual. The information given here is designed to help you make informed decisions about your health. It is not intended as a substitute for any treatment that may have been prescribed by your doctor. If you suspect that you have a medical problem, we urge you to seek competent medical help.

Library of Congress Cataloging-in-Publication Data

Davis, Julie, date.
    Young skin for life : your guide to smoother, clearer, more beautiful skin—at any age / by Julie Davis and the editors of Prevention magazine.
       p.   cm.
    Includes index.
    ISBN 0–87596–240–8 hardcover
    ISBN 0–87596–241–6 paperback
    1. Skin—Care and hygiene.   I. Prevention Magazine Health Books.
II. Title.
RL87.D38   1995
646.7'26—dc20   94-39304

Distributed in the book trade by St. Martin's Press

2 4 6 8 10 9 7 5 3 1   hardcover
2 4 6 8 10 9 7 5 3 1   paperback

———————— OUR MISSION ————————

We publish books that empower people's lives.

—— RODALE 🌱 BOOKS ——

Young Skin for Life Editorial and Design Staff

Managing Editor: **Sharon Faelten**
Editor: **Julia Hansen**
Researchers: **Susan E. Burdick, Carlotta Cuerdon, Christine Dreisbach, Deborah Pedron, Sally A. Reith, Anita Small, Bernadette Sukley**
Studio Manager: **Joe Golden**
Cover Designer: **Faith Hague**
Book Designer: **Lynn N. Gano**
Cover Photographer: **Mark Scott**
Page Layout: **Mary Brundage**
Copy Editors: **Stacey Ann Cortese, Jane Sherman**
Manufacturing Coordinator: **Melinda B. Rizzo**
Office Staff: **Roberta Mulliner, Julie Kehs, Bernadette Sauerwine, Mary Lou Stephen**

PREVENTION Magazine Health Books

Editor-in-Chief, Rodale Books: **Bill Gottlieb**
Executive Editor: **Debora A. Tkac**
Art Director: **Jane Colby Knutila**
Research Manager: **Ann Gossy Yermish**
Copy Manager: **Lisa D. Andruscavage**

For my beautiful daughter,
Alexandra:
eyes of blue,
skin of alabaster,
SPF 30 every day!

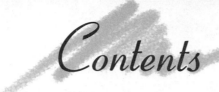

Contents

PART TWO: A Guide to Cosmetics and Skin-Care Products

PART THREE: Nutritional Maintenance for Beautiful Skin

PART FOUR: Quick and Easy Daily Routines for Your Skin Type

Foreword

As organs go, skin certainly suffers its share of problems. A major dermatology textbook describes over 2,000 possible skin diseases! While few skin ailments are deadly or disabling, many are annoying, uncomfortable and unsightly. Skin disorders can have a psychological component as well: They can weaken self-confidence, complicate social and sexual relations and demand a burdensome amount of time and effort to control.

As we grow older, we're more prone to skin disorders. After age 70, most otherwise healthy people will develop at least one skin problem worthy of medical attention, and as many as 20 percent may develop three to five such ailments, be it a mild case of dermatitis, very dry skin or new or deeper wrinkles. As the population ages, skin problems will become the rule rather than the exception.

There are not nearly enough dermatologists to provide professional care for the population at large. The good news is, many common disorders of the skin, hair and nails can be effectively treated at home. But self-treating these conditions safely and successfully requires that certain guidelines be followed. First, correctly identify the condition, as misidentification can have serious consequences. Second, pursue sensible, sound treatment. Many safe and useful products are available in drugstores, but you have to know what works and why. And you have to be able to know when to abandon attempts at self-care and get medical advice.

That is where this book comes in. *Young Skin for Life* is an extremely practical, comprehensive guide to skin care that will enable you to keep your skin healthy and attractive for years to come. The author has sought out the recommendations of over 50 well-known dermatologists, so you can be confident that the remedies you'll find in these pages are based on medical science, not folklore. The writing is clear, concise and lively, and free of medical jargon and unrealistic promises of instant cures.

At a time when people are being urged to take charge of their health, *Young Skin for Life* is a valuable tool.

—**Albert M. Kligman, M.D., Ph.D.**

PART ONE

A Troubleshooting Guide for Common Skin Problems

CHAPTER ONE

Age Spots and Freckles

How to Give Them the Fade

A sprinkling of freckles across a little girl's nose is cute—but you're not a kid anymore. Besides, you're not exactly sure what those little brown splotches on your face, hands or forearms might be. Are they a few renegade freckles, or—ugh—age spots? Whatever they are, you want them to go away.

Not to worry. Getting rid of either of these spotty skin conditions, or at least improving their appearance, can be simple and virtually painless. Read on to find out how.

Taking Aim at Age Spots

These hyperpigmented patches (solar lentigines) range from light brown to black and are usually called age or liver spots. But they have little to do with your age (and nothing to do with your liver). Their primary cause is overexposure to the sun: Age spots pop up when your beleaguered dermis, trying to protect itself from those burning rays, increases its production of melanin, the substance that gives your skin its pigment.

Using a strong sunscreen with a sun protection factor (SPF) of at least 15 is the best way to keep age spots at bay and your skin looking youthful. And while it's never too late to start reaching for the sun-

Picking Out Trouble Spots

Before a dermatologist recommends a treatment for age spots, he or she may want to evaluate the pigmented patches to make sure they're just a cosmetic problem.

Run-of-the-mill age spots can look like spots that may or may not be precancerous, "and they can't easily be differentiated even by experts," says Albert M. Kligman, M.D., Ph.D.

Even the best, most skilled, best-trained dermatologist can find it difficult to tell whether or not a spot is precancerous by just looking at it, says Laurence M. David, M.D., president of the International Society of Cosmetic Laser Surgeons and chief of laser surgery at the Institute of Cosmetic and Laser Surgery in Hermosa Beach, California. "As a general rule, every spot should be biopsied," he says.

It's also a good idea to have your doctor perform a "spot check" as part of your annual physical. And any spot that appears suddenly, bleeds or changes color or shape should be examined further.

glasses or pulling on the gloves, age spots probably won't fade on their own, even if you stop sun-worshiping and start using sunscreens.

So check into "spot treatments" that can lighten or even get rid of age spots entirely. The two main options: over-the-counter and prescription topical (applied directly to the skin) agents and removal by such methods as peeling, freezing or laser treatment. Medical removal, which is performed by a dermatologist, can work faster than the long-term topical treatments, but it tends to be more expensive.

One point bears emphasis: Avoiding the sun and using a strong sunscreen are essential both during and after some of these treatments. They can leave the skin even more vulnerable to the sun.

Bleaching Creams: Do-It-Yourself Spot Removers

You might first try to fade age spots with an over-the-counter bleaching cream formulated with hydroquinone, a chemical that hinders melanin production. But it may not do the job, according to Albert M. Kligman, M.D., Ph.D. "None of these bleaching creams works very well—the concentration of hydroquinone is just too low," he says. (Dr. Kligman says that of the brands he's studied, Porcelana works best.)

Not only can these creams leave age spots intact, they can also carry potential side effects resulting from unmonitored, long-term use of hydroquinone, like darkening of the skin. More alarmingly, the chemical has also caused cancer in lab animals. Yet many physicians say these fade creams aren't dangerous. "A cream formulated with 2 percent hydroquinone is very safe," says Dr. Kligman.

The Food and Drug Administration (FDA) isn't so sure, however. Studies are ongoing, and the FDA says hydroquinone is "under review." For now, products are still on the market, but they should be used with caution and for only a few months at the most, according to an FDA spokesperson.

Prescription-Only Bleaches

If after a few months an over-the-counter fade cream hasn't helped erase your age spots, these dermatologist-prescribed topical treatments might do the trick.

Rub spots with Retin-A. Best known as a remedy for acne and wrinkles, Retin-A (topical tretinoin), a form of vitamin A, can significantly lighten or even clear sun-induced age spots. According to one study conducted by the Department of Dermatology at the University of Michigan Medical Center in Ann Arbor, age spots faded slightly after only a month of nightly treatment with 0.1 percent Retin-A and showed even more improvement in less than a year.

Retin-A can cause redness and scaling if the concentration is too strong, so it's important that your treatment be monitored by your dermatologist. Still, "you should use the highest concentration you can tolerate. Peeling is advisable," says Dr. Kligman, the creator of Retin-A.

Double-team Retin-A with a "fade helper." Retin-A plus hydroquinone (the hydroquinone is prescribed in a higher, more effective concentration than what's in over-the-counter bleaching creams) may lighten age spots even faster. "Retin-A does more by itself than the formulas of hydroquinone alone, but together they are more effective," explains James J. Leyden, M.D., professor of dermatology at the University of Pennsylvania School of Medicine in Philadelphia.

Put spots to the acid test. Alpha hydroxy acids (AHAs)—mild acids derived from natural substances like fruit and milk—are the beauty industry's miracle ingredient of the decade. These acids slough off dead cells on the surface of the skin, seem to improve the appearance of fine lines and rough-textured skin and generally "brighten" the complexion.

AHAs also seem to lighten skin discolorations. Research by Eugene J. Van Scott, M.D., clinical professor of dermatology at Hahnemann University School of Medicine in Philadelphia, showed that the twice-daily application of one AHA, lactic acid (available in the prescription product Lac-Hydrin), combined with in-office chemical peels (see below) lightened age spots and helped peel away harmless skin growths.

The degree of improvement varies, however. Some patients using AHAs see results in as little as 60 days, with quite noticeable results after five months. Others may have to wait a year to see any substantial change. It's also important to note that over-the-counter products formulated with AHAs usually contain far weaker concentrations of the acids and, according to Dr. Kligman, "have no effect."

Give age spots the works. Dermatologists sometimes use a combination of substances to get rid of age spots. Elliot Jacobs, M.D., attending surgeon at New York Eye and Ear Infirmary and Cabrini Medical Center and a plastic surgeon in New York City, treats some age spots with both Retin-A and the AHA glycolic acid. Another "topical cocktail": glycolic acid and hydroquinone.

When Creams Don't Cut It: Doctoring Your Spots

If topical treatments don't do the trick, your dermatologist may be able to remove age spots in one or several office visits. Here are some options.

Peel away pigmented patches. Some of the acids that are used in complexion-smoothing chemical peels, like glycolic acid, are also used to treat age spots. A 50 percent salicylic acid ointment peel can remove stubborn brown spots often found on the hands and forearms, says James M. Swinehart, M.D., medical director of the Denver Dermatology Center.

To help the skin soak up the ointment, Dr. Swinehart has patients pretreat spots with Retin-A for a few weeks or months and performs a mild (20 percent strength) peel with a chemical called tri-chloroacetic acid (TCA) immediately before applying the salicylic acid. The ointment is left on the area, which is bandaged, for two days. The spots start blistering and peeling in two days and clear in about ten days; redness follows for a few more weeks.

Dr. Swinehart believes this method works better than Retin-A or a TCA peel alone. The salicylic acid does occasionally produce tempo-rary side effects, like ringing in the ears and/or muffled hearing within a few hours of its application or a slight burning sensation for a day or two. "This is a high concentration of salicylic acid paste," notes Dr. Kligman, so be prepared for a moderate amount of dis-comfort.

A single treatment (at an average cost of $350) can produce good results, but depending on the severity of the spot, you might need to return for one or more peels.

Freeze out age spots. If you have a history of sensitive skin or if topical treatments haven't helped, freezing spots with liquid nitro-gen may work. Freezing can also be part of a combination therapy. Says Dr. Leyden, "It's not uncommon for someone to have different kinds of lesions—black, dark brown and a variety of others less pig-mented," he says. "I'll usually freeze a couple and have the patient start using Retin-A and hydroquinone on the others."

Pain is surprisingly minimal (15 or 20 seconds of smarting or sting-ing). Dr. Leyden starts with a "light" freeze, which produces only a mild peeling. "I'm more willing to treat a second time if needed," he says.

Freezing age spots does pose some risks, however. According to Laurence M. David, M.D., president of the International Society of Cosmetic Laser Surgeons and chief of laser surgery at the Institute of Cosmetic and Laser Surgery in Hermosa Beach, California, the pro-cedure can cause scarring or remove too much melanin, leaving a white spot where the brown spot used to be.

Zap the patches away. Using laser treatment on age spots "de-stroys the cells making the excess pigmentation, then new, normally functioning pigment cells move back into that area," says Joseph G. Morelli, M.D., assistant professor of dermatology and pediatrics at the University of Colorado School of Medicine in Denver. This method "works best on big, isolated brown spots or on people who have relatively normal skin with just a few obvious spots," he explains.

Laser treatment is generally not painful. Dr. Morelli describes the discomfort as a little pinch or sting during the millionth-of-a-second zap and minor irritation for a half-hour afterward. The area will be discolored at first; within a week, the spot will flake off. The number of treatments necessary varies—one to three for a big brown facial spot and two to five for multiple spots on the hands, in Dr. Morelli's experience. Most doctors space treatments one to two months apart to allow for healing and to determine how much pigment is left.

Dr. Morelli believes laser treatment carries the least risk of scarring or hypopigmentation. On the down side, zapping the spot can be expensive. Dr. David says the price of removal depends on a number of factors, including the spot's size and location. "The cost can range anywhere from a couple hundred dollars to several hundred dollars," he says. Another limitation of the laser: It won't remove raised spots.

Specialists are currently using several different types of lasers to remove age spots—carbon dioxide lasers, ruby lasers and pulsed-dye lasers, among others—and which laser works best is the subject of much debate. One thing is clear, however: Using lasers safely and effectively takes a lot of skill. If you opt for laser treatment, you should, at the very least, find out if your doctor is a member of the American Society for Laser Medicine and Surgery.

CHAPTER TWO

Blemishes

Clearing, Calming Skin Strategies

*P*imples, zits, blemishes—call them what you will, the bumps and blotches associated with acne are distressing with a capital *D*!

Why do some of us break out while others don't? Experts aren't sure. What they do know is that acne results from a complex interaction of factors, including genetic predisposition, hormones that cause the sebaceous (oil) glands to enlarge and excessive oil production.

Acne can be aggravated by factors outside the body, too. The oils in some skin creams or cosmetics can block pores, triggering pimples (but less so than you may think). Stress can also be a factor, especially in women whose acne first flares up after their teens.

While experts don't understand exactly why adult skin sometimes reverts to adolescent behavior, they know how blemishes form. Your skin is constantly renewing itself, and under normal conditions, dead horny cells surface and shed. But when, instead, these cells stick together, they plug the hair follicle, forming what's called a comedone. "Open" comedones are commonly known as blackheads; the "closed" variety, whiteheads. When a closed comedone ruptures, you get a pimple.

Pimples also vary in size and appearance. Papules are tender pimples that look like reddish bumps. Pustules are pimples that have "come to a head." Deep cysts are inflamed "bubbles" that contain blood and pus and can cause scarring. If you have severe blemishes and enlarged blood vessels around the nose, chin or cheeks and you flush or blush easily, see a dermatologist: You may have rosacea (pronounced ro-ZAY-shuh), a skin condition that looks like acne but isn't.

Your antiblemish strategy will depend on what kind of blemish (or blemishes) you have. But no matter which type of pimples you're facing, a dermatologist can help clear up the problem with a variety of very effective treatments.

The Breakout Blues: Not Just for Teens

As mentioned, the end of adolescence doesn't automatically mean the end of blemishes. In fact, some women who remained acne-free during their teens may find themselves facing flare-ups for the first time as adults. Albert M. Kligman, M.D., Ph.D., divides adult acne into two categories: postadolescent and postmenopausal.

Postadolescent acne, which predominantly affects career women in their twenties, thirties and forties (often just before their periods), is stress-induced—fueled by the pressures of juggling career, family and relationships. Postmenopausal acne, hitting in the fifties or beyond, may be influenced by a hormonal imbalance caused by reduced estrogen production.

Both types of "late-blooming acne" usually involve whiteheads and a few scattered blemishes and are more likely to affect women with darker or oily skin (or, in postmenopausal women, with formerly oily skin and large pores) who did not have acne in their teens.

While not serious, either kind of acne is exasperating. But over-the-counter topical treatments (applied directly to the skin) or dermatologist-prescribed medications can go a long way toward restoring a woman's complexion to its youthful clarity.

Benzoyl Peroxide: An On-Your-Own Blemish Blocker

For mild acne, dermatologists often recommend an over-the-counter solution, gel or soap formulated with benzoyl peroxide (available in 2.5, 5 or 10 percent formulas), which kills *P. acnes*, the bacteria that cause acne. Apply to clean, dry skin and only on the blemish itself. The antibacterial action of a full-strength product will produce a mild peeling. But kinder, gentler formulas, with a lower concentration of benzoyl peroxide and timed-release action, can work just as effectively without overdrying or irritating your skin.

Be aware, however, that some people (about 1 out of 20, according to one doctor's estimate), are extremely sensitive to benzoyl peroxide in any amount. Their skin reddens and swells after use. If that happens to you, discontinue using this product immediately.

Rx Relief

If you can't zap blemishes with drugstore medications, consider seeing a dermatologist. Here are some of the most effective treatments available.

Banish blemishes with Retin-A. Though best known as a medical weapon against wrinkles, Retin-A (topical tretinoin) was originally developed by Dr. Kligman to treat acne. The active ingredient in Retin-A, vitamin A, works by expelling the blackheads and whiteheads from which pimples develop. For postmenopausal acne, Dr. Kligman recommends Retin-A in a cream base. "It's better tolerated by mature skin than a solution or gel," he says, and you'll see results in four to six months.

If your blemishes are more severe, your dermatologist may have you use Retin-A at night and benzoyl peroxide in the morning. Used in tandem, they can be more effective than either one alone. *Never* apply them at the same time; benzoyl peroxide can oxidize and inactivate the Retin-A.

Take them out with topical antibiotics. While applying an antibiotic like clindamycin or erythromycin directly to the skin doesn't work quite as well as taking oral antibiotics, says Dr. Kligman (and topical antibiotics take longer to work, from four to six weeks), they have one important advantage: They have fewer side effects than oral antibiotics, which can cause upset stomach, vaginal infections and other problems.

Combining topical antibiotics with other treatments is yet another way to tackle acne. Lawrence Schachner, M.D., of the University of Miami School of Medicine in Florida, found that a mix of erythromycin and zinc acetate (a skin protectant that also helps heal wounds) helped prevent comedones from forming and decreased bacteria and inflammatory lesions. Another effective combination: erythromycin formulated with benzoyl peroxide, or benzamycin.

The erythromycin also lessens the irritating effects of the benzoyl peroxide.

Hit pimples with alpha hydroxy acids (AHAs). These acids, derived from fruit, vegetables and sugar cane, act as exfoliants (which slough off dead skin cells) and are being used to rejuvenate skin. But they can also work on acne. When used under a doctor's supervision, "AHAs can be extraordinarily effective in the prevention and treatment of acne," notes Eugene J. Van Scott, M.D., clinical professor of dermatology at Hahnemann University School of Medicine in Philadelphia. "Stronger solutions can be left on for varying periods of time, then washed off."

Solutions vary from 5 to 70 percent strength. The stronger the solution, the less time it's left on the skin. Generally, AHAs are applied every two to four weeks. Your treatment program will depend on how your skin responds.

Some dermatologists also give their patients AHA products to use at home. But not all dermatologists advocate this added step.

Dr. Van Scott also recommends that you resist self-treating blemishes with over-the-counter AHA formulations without a doctor's supervision. "There are going to be products that haven't undergone preclinical or premarketing testing," he says. "And the acid concentration is so low that they probably won't have much effect." (Although the manufacturers of these preparations aren't required to divulge how much of the acid their products contain, it's usually between 2 and 12 percent.)

Help for Severe Acne

Mild acne is distressing enough; severe acne is cause for anguish. If your acne is serious, don't give up! Chances are you and your dermatologist will be able to work out an effective strategy using one of various treatment plans.

Serious medicine for serious acne. "For severe acne, oral antibiotics like tetracycline are still a mainstay," said Dr. Van Scott. To lessen the side effects of these drugs, some physicians prescribe a lower dosage in combination with a topical medication like Retin-A, a topical antibiotic or both (although not all doctors opt for the latter). Taking tetracycline tends to make you exquisitely vulnerable to the sun, so make sure you always protect your skin with a strong sunscreen with an SPF of at least 15. But don't take tetracycline if you're pregnant or think you might be. This drug can discolor the teeth of children while they're still in the womb.

A minishot of steroids. Dermatologists can also shrink cysts with a shot of an anti-inflammatory corticosteroid. "If you have a large area of inflammation, the best treatment is to inject a small amount of a corticosteroid. It stops the inflammation very quickly," says James J. Leyden, M.D., professor of dermatology at the University of Pennsylvania School of Medicine in Philadelphia.

Take aim with Accutane. The oral counterpart of Retin-A, Accutane (isotretinoin) is reserved for severe acne that does not respond to topical or other oral medications. Accutane shrinks the sebaceous glands and suppresses oil production, cutting off the stuff that fuels pimples and cysts. What's more, it may continue to help even after you stop taking it months later, when oil production has returned to normal.

But this drug can cause a number of significant side effects, including peeling skin; red, irritated eyelids; and parched, inflamed lips. Most alarmingly, Accutane is associated with birth defects. So women (including teens) should not take this drug unless they're 100 percent certain that there's no chance they are pregnant or will conceive within 30 days of stopping treatment with Accutane.

As for what not to do, a few dermatologists still prescribe certain types of birth control pills for severe acne, but it's rare. "Too often, the Pill works at first, then becomes ineffective," explains Dr. Kligman.

Also, Dr. Leyden cautions against having inflamed cysts drained to ward off scarring—a treatment some dermatologists still use. "If you open a lesion, you run the high risk of leaving a slitlike mark that never disappears," he says.

Finally, topical corticosteroids, oral iodine preparations and certain types of oral contraceptives can cause acne. So tell your dermatologist about any medications other doctors have prescribed for you.

How to Break Out of the Breakout Trap

Whether you're faced with a tiny pimple on your chin or a full-fledged flare-up, these strategies can help you attain clearer, smoother skin (or convincingly camouflage what you can't get rid of).

Stop the rough stuff. Treat your skin gently—no picking, squeezing or scrubbing, no matter how great the temptation! "Compulsive washing and scrubbing worsen acne," warns Dr. Kligman. Contrary to what many people think, aggressive cleansing won't reduce oil production. Quite the contrary: Vigorous scrubbing may generate more oil.

Lose the goop. It's okay to camouflage blemishes with tinted acne medications, but avoid heavy, oil-based skin creams and makeups: Some oils used in cosmetics are comedogenic, meaning they block pores and give rise to blemishes. While Dr. Kligman agrees that certain cosmetics can induce or aggravate acne, "their role has been grossly exaggerated," he maintains. Still, you may be better off using products labeled noncomedogenic, which don't contain oil or other acne-triggering ingredients.

"Feed" your skin right. There's no hard evidence to link breakouts with eating fatty foods like chocolate, pizza, nuts and potato chips, but they won't promote a peaches-and-cream complexion, either.

Conceal the evidence. Even a fading pimple can be bothersome. "As they go away, all pimples—particularly highly inflamed ones—leave behind a flat red mark that can last for months," says Dr. Leyden. "People often mistake these blemishes for scars. But real scars are depressed—like chickenpox—or take the form of small, raised bumps."

Until the marks eventually fade—and they will—you might use a green-tinted cover-up on the spot, suggests Dr. Kligman. (Yes, green!) These concealers won't look green on your face, though; they'll simply "cancel out" the color of the mark. (Green counteracts red.) You can find the cover-ups at a good pharmacy or the cosmetics area of a large department store or mall.

Note: While most makeup artists believe tinted bases look fake when they're worn over the entire face to "correct" skin tone, they are an option for spot relief.

Try a serious superconcealer. If you need more than spot coverage, Laura Geller, makeup artist and owner of Laura Geller Make-Up Studios, a cosmetics store in New York City, recommends Derma Color, a stage makeup that provides great camouflage.

See also the chapters on concealers (chapter 23), acne-prone skin (chapter 42), collagen (chapter 46), dermabrasion (chapter 48) and Retin-A (chapter 51).

CHAPTER THREE

Blisters, Calluses and Corns

Relief for Feet under Pressure

*I*f one of Cinderella's stepsisters had managed to squeeze her feet into those tiny glass slippers, she could have ended up with more than the handsome prince—a blister, a callus or even a corn or two!

It just goes to prove that pretty shoes aren't necessarily comfortable ones. In fact, repeated friction and pressure from ill-fitting shoes are the main cause of all three of these common—and often painful—foot problems. When shoes are too snug, the top layer of skin toughens and thickens to protect tender skin from the constant chafing. If the friction continues, you'll get a corn or a callus. (It depends on where your tough shoe is meeting tender skin.) Add heat or dampness to the friction, and you get a blister—a painful, fluid-filled tear within the skin's layers.

These annoying foot ailments can also have a domino effect. "If one part of your foot constantly gets blisters, it will frequently become callused and may ultimately develop a corn," says Glenn Gastwirth, D.P.M., deputy executive director of the American Podiatric Medical Association in Bethesda, Maryland.

There are two kinds of corns: hard and soft. Hard corns usually form on the top of the little toe. The soft kind prefers the moist atmosphere found between your toes. Whether a corn is hard or soft depends on how much sweat it's exposed to.

Is Your Workout Fit for Your Feet?

An hour into your workout, you're starting to feel the burn. Unfortunately, it's situated in your feet! These tips can keep you on your toes—without pain.

Give yourself some space. Make sure your toes aren't slamming into the front of your aerobic shoes while you exercise. "You want a thumb's-width of space between your big toe and the end of the shoe," says Michael L. Ramsey, M.D., clinical instructor of dermatology at Baylor College of Medicine in Houston. "If you feel soreness on the sides of or in between your toes, get a shoe with a wider toe box."

Don't get sore. To keep corns away, cover friction-prone areas, like your little toe or heel, with adhesive bandages. Or use a runner's trick: Just stick a piece of adhesive tape over the sore spot. You might try UltraThon Foam Tape from 3M, a thin, lightweight tape that stays secure through heavy workouts. Protect a callus on the bottom of your foot with insoles. "Buy a pair of insoles, cut out a hole that corresponds to the callused area, and put it in the shoe," suggests Dr. Ramsey.

Keep your feet dry. Dampness encourages blisters, so let shoes

By contrast, a callus is broader than a corn, and you can get calluses on your fingers and palms if you work with your hands a lot. A callus also lacks the distinguishing feature of a corn—a hard "core"—and often shows up on the balls and sides of the feet, around the heel and the tops of the toes. Calluses are just as annoying as corns, but they're usually not painful.

It's easy to see why the feet are on the receiving end of all these problems. First, they carry you and all your weight around each day. "Repeated steps mean repeated friction," says Dr. Gastwirth. And as great as it is for the rest of you, exercise, particularly high-impact aerobics, puts even more pressure on your feet. Finally, factor in the natural bodily changes that occur as we get older. Feet often swell from circulatory changes, spread out a little as the ligaments and muscles that support the body weaken and lose some of their protective fatty padding.

dry out between wearings and have a backup pair in case they get wet. Also, sprinkle powder in your shoes to cut down on chafing. If your feet perspire heavily during exercise, think about changing into dry footwear midway through your workout. And during the summer, Dr. Ramsey also suggests exercising in the early morning or at night, when it's coolest.

Look for leather steppers. If you can, buy leather or canvas athletic footwear; they let feet breathe better than man-made materials. But if your shoes aren't leather or canvas, that's okay—just wear good thick socks to absorb perspiration. You might try Thor-Lo socks. They're made of acrylic, which works better than cotton or wool to help wick away blister-breeding moisture, but they're thick, so wear them while you're trying on a new pair of athletic shoes; they may make a snug fit painfully snug.

Break in new footwear gradually. Keep blisters at bay by wearing new aerobic shoes around the house before lacing them up for a full workout. For example, "if you normally run ten miles, run in the new shoes for three miles, then move up to six, then go the full ten," says Dr. Ramsey.

But tough or blistered feet can respond quickly to tender loving care. In fact, after following these foot "steps," you may even splurge on a new pair of sandals for prettier (and pain-free) feet!

Step 1: Lose the Cruel Shoes

Throwing out shoes that hurt is the first step in banishing blisters and thickened skin, so peruse your shoes (and hose) for the prime suspects of pain.

Shoe fit. Are your shoes too tight? Too loose? Either can cause blisters, calluses and corns. Try having tight footwear stretched to stop the chafing. This won't work, though, if the shoes have seams that press on the painful area.

Shoe design. A too-shallow, narrow or pointy toe box (the front part of your shoe) pressing against your little toe can cause a hard corn. A too-snug toe box might also mash toes together, forming a between-the-toe soft corn. Too high a heel counter—the part of the shoe that surrounds the back of the heel—promotes blisters and thickened skin, as do straps that rub and chafe your foot or ankle.

Shoe condition. Look for loose or unevenly stitched seams or tears in the linings of your shoes. They can create rough edges that rub against your heel or ankle.

Hosiery design or condition. Wearing socks with worn-out heels or holes or stockings that wad up at the toe or heel promotes blisters. So does heavy stitching across the toe of a sock.

Step 2: Get Shoe Savvy

Your snazzy new shoes felt fine in the store. Now you're wincing with every step you take! Try these tips the next time you buy.

Let professionals fit you. Sometimes it's hard to find the shoe that fits: One company's size 9, for example, can be roomier or tighter than another's. So shop shoe stores staffed with trained salespeople. They'll be able to measure your feet correctly, recommend wider or narrower styles and generally help you find shoes that fit like they're supposed to. But steer clear of the salesperson who insists that a 9AA shoe fits your 8½B foot.

Don't force the issue. Don't try to jam your feet into shoes that are even a half-size too small (even if they're on sale). The same rule applies even if you're trying on the size you've been wearing for years. "Feet spread as we get older," explains Dr. Gastwirth, so growing into a larger size is perfectly natural.

And since one foot is usually slightly wider or longer (or both) than the other, size shoes to that foot (a salesperson will be able to help with this). The store can give you a little pad to put in the other one.

Don't stretch shoes to the "breaking-in" point. Properly fitted shoes are not quite snug and definitely not tight. For dress shoes, allow about a half-inch between your big toe and the tip of the shoe. Don't fool yourself into believing that they'll stretch out eventually—you can't break in the wrong size. "If they feel bad when you put them on, they're probably going to get worse, not better," says Michael L. Ramsey, M.D., clinical instructor of dermatology at Baylor College of Medicine in Houston.

Purchase in the P.M. Try to buy shoes (particularly heels) in the late afternoon or at night. Your feet can swell by a full size or more by the end of the day.

Have the right hose on hand. It seems obvious, but try on sneakers with socks, heels with panty hose.

Become "well-heeled." High heels are a prime cause of blisters, calluses and corns and can also contribute to the development of back problems. But if you're determined to "walk tall," take steps to limit the damage.

"Keep your time in heels to a minimum," advises Dr. Ramsey. "When in transit to the office, wear jogging shoes; when you're sitting at your desk, kick off your shoes and wiggle your toes." And if you'll be wearing heels at night, wear flat shoes during the day.

You might also try the lower-heeled (but still stylish) "comfort heels," like those from Easy Spirit. They have a wider toe box, more cushioning in the sole (primarily around the ball of the foot—right where you need it when you wear heels) and more shock absorption, which acts as a buffer between hard pavement and soft foot.

Step 3: Remedy the Pain

Have your feet already paid the price of being fashionable? Then stop the pain—and blisters, calluses and corns—cold, with these simple remedies.

Blister relief. There aren't many things more painful than a blister, but you can get quick relief. Of course, the best treatment is prevention.

To keep blisters from popping up in the first place, create a buffer zone to protect tender spots against chafing. Smear the blister-prone area with petroleum jelly or precushion it with moleskin, a thin adhesive felt you'll find in the foot-care section of most drugstores. Also, powder your feet to fend off dampness and reduce rubbing.

If it's practical, try blister-proofing your feet by wearing two pairs of socks. That way, the sock rubs against another sock, not against your skin. One brand to try: the Thor-Lo line of sports-specific socks available in sporting goods stores. Their extra cushioning can help relieve friction and pressure. You might also wear them for workouts.

You probably already know how to get rid of a blister—you pop it. But there is a right way to do it. Here's how: Clean the blister with alcohol or peroxide. After sterilizing a needle with alcohol or over a flame, prick the blister on the fluid-filled side. Apply gentle pressure to drain the fluid, but don't remove its "roof"—it protects the blister from infection. Apply antibiotic ointment and cover with gauze or an adhesive bandage. Don't use moleskin—it'll stick to the blister.

Think before You Cut!

You have a thick, ugly callus on your heel and you want to get rid of it. Who ya gonna call?

In some cases, the spa or salon. But be careful: While a trained aesthetician is qualified to remove superficial dead skin, never let him or her attempt to treat a serious callus. This procedure requires medical attention, says Glenn Gastwirth, D.P.M., deputy executive director of the American Podiatric Medical Association in Bethesda, Maryland.

Even if your callus-smoothing treatment will be purely cosmetic, it's extremely important to make sure that the tools used are properly sterilized. So before you shed a sock, Dr. Gastwirth recommends that you ask the aesthetician about sterilization procedures.

Also, people with diabetes or poor circulation should have corns or calluses cut away only by a doctor. This lessens the chance of infection.

If the blister's already ruptured and part of the roof is off, just clean it with peroxide, apply the ointment and stick on a bandage.

What to do for calluses. If you're simply looking for relief, moleskin or shock-absorbing Spenco insoles, made of a cushiony, rubber-like material, will pad painful calluses. If you want to actually get rid of the thickened skin, try a nightly buffing with a pumice stone, an abrasive stone used to slough off dead skin. They're available at drugstores. Here's how: Clean and soften your callus in warm soapy water for 10 to 15 minutes. Then rub the pumice stone back and forth across the callus—*gently*. "A pumice stone can create an abrasion on healthy skin," says Dr. Ramsey. "Buff gently and slowly, stop, then decide whether to keep going."

The longer you've had the callus, the longer it will take to get rid of it, so be patient and keep up the soak-and-buff routine. Never try to cut away a callus yourself—let a doctor do it.

Coping with corns. To ease the pressure and provide temporary relief, cushion corns with nonmedicated moleskin or corn pads. To relieve the throb of a soft corn, put a piece of lamb's-wool, moleskin or cotton or a corn pad between your toes. The doughnut-shaped corn pads may also help, but the hole has to line up with the corn.

Actually removing corns is harder. Try a nightly buffing with a pumice stone. Never try to cut away a corn yourself.

Think twice about trying those over-the-counter corn removers, however. They're usually formulated with salicylic acid, which can eat right through the corn to the tender skin underneath, and many doctors don't recommend their use. Salicylic acid removers (and the medicated corn pads) are especially dangerous for people with diabetes or poor circulation. People with these health conditions are less able to fight off infections. And because they often lose feeling in their feet, they may not notice a budding or even an advanced infection. If you have diabetes or circulatory problems, experts say not to use these products and to have the corn professionally removed.

Actually, having a podiatrist pare away your corn may be the best way to go, especially if it's extremely painful or isn't responding to self-treatment. "A podiatrist can remove corns and calluses fairly painlessly and take measures that can keep them from coming back," says Dr. Ramsey.

When to Get Professional Help

Head to a podiatrist, also called a doctor of podiatric medicine, if your corn or callus is extremely painful or you think it may be infected, which is possible if you tried to cut it away yourself. Signs of infection include redness, swelling or pus formation.

A podiatrist can find out exactly what's causing your problem—and can usually offer a simple solution. "The earlier something is taken care of, the easier it is to treat," says Dr. Ramsey.

If the way you walk is causing your corns, for example, a podiatrist can correct your gait with orthotics. These customized shoe inserts, made from a cast of your foot, can ease the pain of corns or calluses. She might also recommend you wear special shoes with cutouts on the inside along the areas of chronic friction. They'll ease painful pressure and distribute your weight more evenly.

If your footwear isn't causing the problem, your doctor may suggest surgery to fix the underlying cause of corns or calluses. "If you're dealing with a toe disfigurement, it's best treated by correcting the deformity, rather than constantly treating the symptoms," says Dr. Gastwirth. Surgery isn't always necessary, he notes, "but it may be an option if other treatment methods don't work."

CHAPTER FOUR

Bruises

First-Aid for the Black and Blues

The phone's ringing as you let yourself in your front door. Racing into the kitchen, you turn the corner of your desk too fast and—*ouch!*—jab your thigh against its sharp edge. Muttering under your breath, you reach for the receiver, trying to ignore the pain and resigning yourself to a large bruise the color of Concord grapes. Adding insult to injury, you missed your call!

Bruises are nature's technicolor response to blunt trauma as blood vessels beneath the skin surface leak into surrounding tissue, turning your skin black or gray at first, then a rainbow of blues, purples, greens and yellows. It takes several days—sometimes weeks—for your body to reabsorb this blood, which is why the discoloration stays . . . and stays . . . and stays!

Whether you're 6 or 60, black-and-blue marks aren't pretty. But if you act right away, you can minimize their swelling and tenderness.

Act Fast with Ice

Cryotherapy is a formal term for applying ice (or anything cold) to injuries to soft tissues like muscles, joints and ligaments. And ice is a safe, easy and effective remedy for bruises. Slapping an "ice bandage" on a black-and-blue mark as soon as possible helps minimize a bruise by constricting the blood vessels, helping to control bleeding within the muscle. The less bleeding, the smaller the bruise.

Ice minimizes a bruise in other ways, too. "It calms down the inflammatory reaction, so you're going to see a quicker decrease in the swelling," says Michael L. Ramsey, M.D., clinical instructor of dermatology at Baylor College of Medicine in Houston. "Getting rid of the inflammation will lessen the pain as well."

This Plant Helps Heal Bruises

Centuries ago, people used the flowering plant mountain arnica to treat muscle pain and soreness. Today, some doctors recommend arnica in gel or tablet form to help cut the pain, swelling and possibly the unsightliness of bruises.

George Fareed, M.D., who specializes in sports medicine at Pioneers Medical Center in Brawley, California, suggests arnica gel to his patients with sports injuries. "Arnica is soothing and has a local anti-inflammatory effect that can speed up the healing process," he says.

Apply arnica gel to a bruise two to four times a day, suggests Dr. Fareed. "Massage it in until it's absorbed and the area is dry." The average bruise will fade in two to four days, he says, "considerably less time than if left to heal on its own." You may even find your bruise skips the black-and-blue stage altogether and goes straight to a very light yellow.

Arnica isn't only used to treat run-of-the-mill bruises. Marjorie Cramer, M.D., clinical assistant professor of surgery at St. Vincent's Hospital in New York City and owner of the Cramer Center for Cosmetic Surgery, suggests her patients try arnica tablets to help reduce postoperative swelling and bruising.

You can find arnica gel and tablets at health food stores and drugstores that sell homeopathic products. But whichever product you try, follow the instructions on the label and don't take more than the recommended amount in the hopes of speedier results. Even medicinal herbs are potent stuff.

Ice works best when applied immediately, so don't wait: Any way you ice down the bruise will help, says Dr. Ramsey. You should apply "cold comfort" at least three times a day for 15 minutes each time. "More often would be ideal, but it's not always practical. Most people can't afford to be sitting around with ice packs on all day!" adds Dr. Ramsey. Just about the only thing ice therapy won't do is eliminate discoloration. Unless you can cover a bruise with concealer, you'll just have to wait out its natural progression from purple to green to yellow, until it fades on its own.

Caution: If you are overly sensitive or insensitive to cold or are allergic to cold, don't try ice therapy without first talking to your doctor. And don't ice a bruise if you have Raynaud's disease. People with Raynaud's disease or any other sensitivity to cold may not know when to stop ice therapy and should consult a doctor before applying cold to their skin.

RICE: More Help for Unsightly Smashups

RICE is short for rest, ice, compression and elevation. Add these extras to ice therapy if your bruise is very tender or swollen. "Also choose RICE when the bruise is very painful and when you have the time to rest the area," Dr. Ramsey adds.

Wrapping the bruise with an elastic bandage can cut swelling faster than ice alone and help reabsorb blood and other fluid that's leaked from injured vessels under the skin, explains Dr. Ramsey. Raising the injured area above the level of your heart reduces blood flow to the area and helps bring the swelling down.

RICE works best on the arms and legs, notes Dr. Ramsey. Applying RICE to your thigh right after walking into your desk could prevent deep bruising in the muscle, for example.

On Your Toes: Bruised or Broken?

Say that while stumbling around in the dark on your way to the bathroom, you crack one of your little piggies against the bathtub. Stubbing a toe may be the stuff of TV sitcoms, but it's not funny when it happens to you. And what you think is a minor mishap might actually be quite serious.

According to Glenn Gastwirth, D.P.M., deputy executive director of the American Podiatric Medical Association in Bethesda, Maryland, a stubbed toe that turns black and blue could actually be broken.

In the past, doctors didn't pay too much attention to broken toes, the thinking being that they would heal on their own if you went easy on them for a few days. But that's changed, says Dr. Gastwirth: If you don't get medical help for a broken toe, it may not heal right and could end up deformed.

If your toe looks disfigured, rises a bit higher than other toes or feels limp and loose, it could be broken. So check it out, especially if you also see swelling or feel pinpoint tenderness or throbbing-type pain. Your toe might be dislocated rather than broken. But it still needs medical attention, says Dr. Gastwirth.

Nowadays, doctors fix a broken toe by simply splinting it and taping it to the toe next to it. They'll also tell patients with a fractured tootsie to cut back on their activities for at least a month—maybe longer, depending on how bad the break is. "Rush back into strenuous activities, and a toe that would have healed in four to six weeks may take longer to fix," says Dr. Gastwirth.

While most doctors can treat a broken toe, seeing a podiatrist may be a better choice, because they're more familiar with this type of injury. Seeing a podiatrist is also a good idea because a stress or hairline fracture may not show up on an x-ray right away, and a foot specialist should be able to diagnose a broken toe even without consulting an x-ray.

Another bruised-toe problem that shouldn't be ignored is "tennis toe," which is also called jogger's toe or skier's toe, depending on the sport. When your big toe repeatedly slams against the front of your shoe during the activity (think of your aerobics class), you can get bleeding under the toenail, which can turn the nail black, says Rodney S. W. Basler, M.D., head of a task force on sports medicine and assistant professor of dermatology at the University of Nebraska Medical Center in Omaha. Your toenail might even fall off if the injury is severe enough, leaving the area open to infection.

If you're sidelined by tennis toe, the best treatment is staying off the foot and soaking the toe in warm water. But if the toe starts throbbing, see a podiatrist. He can stop the pain, caused by the pressure of pooled blood, by draining it. And please, no self-surgery!

You can avoid tennis toe altogether by making sure your athletic shoes fit properly. Dr. Basler also suggests keeping toenails short and trimming them straight across to keep them from hitting the front of your shoes.

Why Mature Skin Bruises Easily

A condition common in older women, senile purpura is named for bruises that can sometimes spontaneously appear on the hands, arms and occasionally the legs. Like other bruises, the ailment is caused by bleeding under the skin, says Albert M. Kligman, M.D., Ph.D.

The condition affects only photodamaged, fragile, thin skin, he adds. Because blood vessels can become fragile over the years, the slightest bump will cause a black-and-blue mark. "Because of poor blood circulation, it takes months for the blood to be reabsorbed," adds Dr. Kligman.

Senile purpura isn't dangerous, but it can be unattractive. Try body makeup like Dermablend or Covermark to cover the bruises.

If you have senile purpura, Dr. Kligman recommends that you do your best to avoid bumping and jarring your skin. Applying petroleum jelly to bruise-prone areas can also reduce your chance of bruising, he adds. "It makes the skin sturdier."

Vitamin K: A New Way to KO Bruises?

Doctors have long used injections of vitamin K—used by the body to coagulate blood—to prevent and control excessive bleeding. According to Melvin L. Elson, M.D., medical director of the Dermatology Center in Nashville and co-author of *The Good Look Book*, vitamin K can also help heal bruises—especially those caused by senile purpura—by speeding reabsorption of the blood that leaks into surrounding tissue.

Dr. Elson, creator of a vitamin K cream called Vitamin K Formula, performed a study in which 12 people who had bruises on their arms and hands used the vitamin K cream on one arm and hand and an identical cream—minus the vitamin K—on the other. After a month, the areas treated with the vitamin K cream had fewer bruises than those treated with the placebo cream.

What's more, applying the vitamin K cream before cosmetic or reconstructive surgery helped to reduce bruising, according to studies done in conjunction with cosmetic surgeons. The cream is available through dermatologists and cosmetic surgeons.

See also the chapters on blisters, calluses and corns (chapter 3) and concealers (chapter 23).

CHAPTER FIVE

Burns

Put Out the Fire—Fast

Take a quick inventory of your skin—especially your hands, wrists and face. Does your hide bear the telltale signs of accidental run-ins with scalding tea, hot irons, oven racks and the like? The unfortunate thing about burns is that you often pay twice: once while you endure the pain and unsightliness of the burn and again if you have to live with the scar, which sometimes takes months or years to fade. One woman burned her temple with a curling iron. The angry spot blistered (predictably) and healed (eventually) but left a brown patch that looked exactly like an age spot for about a year.

More than two million people burn themselves in the United States each year. Fortunately, most of these burns are minor—damage inflicted during accidental contact with hot liquids, a heated iron or other metal, flames or caustic chemicals.

Knowing what to do—and doing it fast—can speed healing and greatly minimize chances that a burn will leave a permanent scar.

Burns: A Matter of Degree

Burns are classified as first-, second- or third-degree, depending on how deep the damage is and how much surface area is affected.

A first-degree burn causes little more than superficial damage (a mild sunburn is a good example). It's red and painful but doesn't cause skin loss.

A second-degree burn destroys the skin's outer layer (the epidermis) and some of its inner layer (the dermis), and the burned skin may swell and blister. That's why a severe sunburn causes peeling, but a mild sunburn does not. You can also get a second-degree burn by briefly touching something extremely hot. If you accidentally bump your temple while using a curling iron—or in haste, grab it by the business end—you'll get a second-degree burn. It hurts to the touch and may take a month to heal.

Third-degree burns—caused by longer exposure to heat, flames, chemicals or boiling water—are much worse, destroying the epidermis and the dermis, plus nerves. Since third-degree burns are often life-threatening and need special medical care, this chapter focuses on everyday burns that you can handle on your own.

Skin-Saving Ways to Cool a Burn

The next time you bump into a hot radiator or scald your wrist pouring a cup of tea, try these quick remedies for everyday burns.

Do the big chill. Plunge a minor burn into cold water right away. The cold bath will ease the pain and decrease the chance of skin damage by lowering the temperature of the burned skin. "I'd personally use cold water on a burn because it works so quickly and well," says Robert Sheridan, M.D., director of the Acute Burn Service at the Shriners Burns Institute, staff surgeon in Burn and Trauma Services at Massachusetts General Hospital and assistant professor of surgery at Harvard Medical School, all located in Boston.

Keep your burn submerged for at least a half-hour. The burn's temperature will drop sooner than that, but the longer you keep it cool, the less it will hurt. (Stick a cold pack in your freezer, too. This gel-filled plastic pouch, available in drugstores, doesn't freeze completely and can be "molded" to facial burns or other areas that can't be easily dunked in water.)

Don't use cold water on a very large burn (over both legs, for example). It could cause a condition called total body hypothermia, when your core body temperature drops below normal. "It could be fatal," says John P. Heggers, Ph.D., professor of surgery in the Division of Plastic and Reconstructive Surgery, professor of microbiology at the University of Texas Medical Branch and director of

Simple Cover-Ups for Burn Scars

Whether it's on your face, hand, arm or leg, the scar a burn can leave behind can be troublesome—and regular concealers may not offer as much coverage as you'd like. That's where the Natural Cover line of corrective makeup comes in. These products, created by Linda Seidel, an aesthetic rehabilitation specialist in Baltimore, are made especially to cover burn scars.

You can wear the corrective makeup base (available in eight shades), as a foundation, or you can customize it with one of four corrective makeup tints: There's a pink tint for lighter skin, reddish brown for darker white skin or lighter black skin, deep red for darker black skin and yellow for extremely olive or Asian complexions. The line also includes four shades of corrective powders that seal and waterproof the makeup bases and coversticks (also in four shades) for small scars and quick touch-ups.

clinical microbiology at the Shriners Burns Institute in Galveston.

And never put ice on your burn. Although ice works well for a bruise, it can further damage burned skin.

Say aloe. The gel of the aloe vera plant, a member of the lily family, has been used as a healing agent since Hippocrates' day, according to Dr. Heggers, who has studied aloe vera extensively and firmly believes in its power to heal.

To keep the burn-cooling relief of aloe on hand, consider getting a plant for home. The next time you iron your finger along with your blouse, all you'll have to do is cut a spike from the cactuslike plant and smooth the fluid inside over your burn.

Dr. Heggers also suggests Dermaide Aloe Cream, available in drugstores, which contains 70 percent aloe vera gel. Dr. Heggers found that Dermaide worked even better than aloe vera straight from the plant because it's more concentrated. "The more concentrated it is, the better the burn's response," he says.

Smooth your burn with either pure aloe vera or Dermaide three times a day, even under a bandage if you've chosen to dress or cover the burn (see below).

You can use Dermaide by itself, says Dr. Heggers. But you might want to team it with an antibiotic salve, which helps prevent infection but seems to slow the healing process. Using Dermaide in tandem with a medicated salve, however, may reverse this side effect, according to research done by Dr. Heggers.

Note: Some doctors feel using any other product with an antibiotic ointment weakens the ointment's healing power.

Dress your burn. Even a small burn hurts a lot. Damaged nerve endings are acutely sensitive to the slightest touch. So protecting a burn can reduce pain and keep out dirt.

To dress a burn, first wash it gently. Soap and water is fine. "Don't let your burn dry out or get dirty," says Dr. Sheridan.

Next, apply antibiotic salve. "Keep the burn clean and covered with antibiotic salve, which will lessen the small chance of infection and may also keep the burn moist and comfortable," says Dr. Sheridan. (Burns heal better in a moist environment.) Do not use butter, lard or anything that contains salt, says Dr. Heggers. For a more serious burn, your doctor may prescribe a silver sulfadiazine cream, which contains an antibacterial agent often used to treat burns.

After smoothing on the antibiotic ointment, cover your burn with a sterile nonstick pad (a nonadhesive dressing won't pull your skin when it's changed). Rather than tape the pad directly to your skin, try wrapping a length of stretchable gauze around the dressing once or twice to hold it in place.

Check the healing. Although your burn is under wraps, it's important to keep an eye on how it's healing. "Check your burn every one to two days, sooner if the pain gets worse—that's a sign of early infection," says Dr. Sheridan. In that case, call your doctor.

If your burn blisters, don't pop it—leave it alone, advises Dr. Sheridan. But if the blister is very large, let your doctor decide how to proceed: Some doctors prefer to drain the blister and remove its top, or "roof," to keep bacteria from getting trapped underneath it, while others prefer to preserve the roof so it can lie on top of the wound and act as a natural dressing.

A ripped or leaking blister can be a veritable welcome mat for infection-causing bacteria. "If you have a very small, superficial blister—smaller than the size of a dime—and it doesn't look infected, it's fine to remove it yourself at home," says Dr. Sheridan. Clean a leaking blister with alcohol or iodine and gently remove its roof with scissors whose blades have been dipped in boiling water. Then dress the burn.

Eat to heal. Powering up your eating habits can help heal a burn, experts say. While eating right is more important in the case of severe burns, getting enough vitamins and minerals helps mend minor scorches, too, says Michele Gottschlich, R.D., Ph.D., director of nutrition services at Shriners Burns Institute in Cincinnati.

Save Your Skin!

When you iron, you're careful not to scorch your blouses. Why not show your skin the same consideration? These tips can help keep your skin smooth (and may save more than your hide).

Cool down your hot-water heater. A hot bubble bath can be soothing, but not if it scalds your skin! "The water coming out of the hot tap can be surprisingly hot," says Robert Sheridan, M.D., director of the Acute Burn Service at the Shriners Burns Institute, staff surgeon in Burn and Trauma Services at Massachusetts General Hospital and assistant professor of surgery at Harvard Medical School, all located in Boston. "A one-second exposure at 160°F can cause a severe burn, and many hot-water heaters are set that high."

If you're continually burning yourself with tap water, lower your water heater's temperature to 120° to 125°, recommends Dr. Sheridan.

Burn-proof your kitchen and cooking habits. Don't wear flowing nightgowns or wide sleeves while you're cooking. "And when you handle hot pots and pans, use mitts, which protect your entire hand and wrist, rather than small square pot holders," says Dr. Sheridan.

Slow down, be careful! All too often, people burn themselves because they're in a hurry, not paying attention or trying to do two things at once. If that's your style, pace yourself. Your beautiful skin will be more apt to stay burn-free.

"You don't need to get carried away, but vitamins, minerals and protein are certainly vital to healing small burns, especially vitamins A and C and the mineral zinc. All of these help skin heal and form collagen," says Dr. Gottschlich. You might even add a stress-formula multivitamin/mineral supplement to a nutritious diet filled with fruits and vegetables, breads and grains, lean meat, milk and dairy products like cheese, low-fat yogurt and cottage cheese.

"And be sure to eat enough protein," adds Dr. Gottschlich. "Skin is protein, so you need protein to get that skin to heal." Good sources of protein include lean poultry, nonfat cheeses, lentils or soybeans, peanut butter and tuna.

Try aspirin to ease the pain. If your burn is causing you discomfort, try taking a few aspirin or other over-the-counter painkillers like ibuprofen.

When a Burn Is Too Hot to Handle

As mentioned, you can probably treat most burns at home. But there are a few situations in which you should have a doctor examine your burn.

If your burn is slow to heal. "Usually, a minor burn, like a mild sunburn, stops hurting and goes away quickly within 48 hours," says Dr. Heggers. "If it persists beyond that, definitely see a doctor."

If you think your burn is getting infected. "Although infection is not common, it can occur," Dr. Sheridan notes. Symptoms of the infection, called burn wound cellulitis, include increasing redness around the burn, fever, pus and more, rather than less, pain. The burn may also have a bad odor.

"Be vigilant throughout the healing period," Dr. Sheridan advises. "Infection can occur anywhere from one or two days to two weeks after the burn."

If it's an emergency. "Getting the right care right away can make a huge difference in how well you recover," says Dr. Sheridan. So if you get a burn you know requires serious medical attention, cover it with a dry, nonlinty bandage or pad and head to the emergency room or your doctor's office.

But don't put anything else on your burn: Creams or salves have to be removed when your burn is examined, which can be painful, says Dr. Sheridan.

CHAPTER SIX

Canker Sores and Fever Blisters

How to Stop the Sting

You can't crack a smile, brush your teeth or eat without discomfort: You've got a canker sore. Or is it a fever blister? All you know is, it looks awful—and it hurts.

While canker sores and fever blisters (also called cold sores) are both small and uncomfortable and pop up in or around your mouth, their causes—and cures—are quite different. But you don't have to let either of these irritating sores get you down in the mouth. You can easily soothe their sting and—in most cases—heal them fast.

Putting Out Fire Sores

The medical name for canker sores, aphthous ulcers, literally means fire sores. And these relatively tiny eruptions can make you feel like your mouth is ablaze.

A canker sore begins as a round or oval red area that usually ruptures within a day, leaving a gray patch ringed by a red halo. Some people get canker sores once in a blue moon; others are plagued time and time again. And while you'll most likely escape with only one sore per outbreak, it's possible to reap a bumper crop all over the inside of your mouth, including your lips, tongue, throat and gums.

There's no cure for cankers. But take heart: As people approach middle age, they tend to suffer fewer (if any) attacks.

What's Going On in Your Mouth?

Canker sores are common—experts say one out of five people will get at least one at one time or another. Yet doctors aren't really sure what causes these irritating eruptions.

It's thought that certain foods like nuts and chocolate, or acidic foods, like oranges, may trigger canker sores. Other canker sore triggers may include emotional stress or trauma to your mouth from a dental procedure or from accidentally biting the inside of your cheek while you're chewing. Some women find they're susceptible to canker sores during certain phases of their menstrual cycle.

Not getting enough iron, folate or vitamin B_{12} may account for 10 to 15 percent of all canker sores, according to James F. Rooney, M.D., associate director of the Department of Infectious Diseases and Immunology at Burroughs-Wellcome in Research Triangle Park, North Carolina. So if you get more than your fair share of cankers, consider adding a multivitamin/mineral supplement containing these vitamins and minerals to your diet, suggests Dr. Rooney.

Pay more than lip service to a mouth sore that doesn't heal, however, on the off chance that it might be something more serious. "Any sore that lasts more than two weeks should be checked out by a dentist or a doctor," says Dr. Rooney.

Another Good Reason to Use Lip Block

According to a study conducted by James F. Rooney, M.D., associate director of the Department of Infectious Diseases and Immunology at Burroughs-Wellcome in Research Triangle Park, North Carolina, up to one-quarter of fever blisters are activated by unprotected exposure to the sun. So using a lip balm with added sunscreen and a sun protection factor (SPF) of at least 15 every time you venture outdoors may lessen your chances of developing a sun-induced fever blister. And you can even apply them under lipstick.

Apply the balm about a half-hour before you go out, and reapply it frequently: You can unintentionally wipe out your protection by eating, drinking, licking your lips and talking.

Easy Does It Is the Best Approach

Here's a rundown of the most common over-the-counter canker treatments. Whichever remedy you use, however, give it a chance to work (and give your sore mouth a break) by limiting your diet to bland, easy-to-eat foods like cooked cereal, scrambled eggs and mashed potatoes. And as obvious as it may seem, avoid salty, spicy or tough-to-chew foods and acidic fruits and juices.

Soothe a sore with gel. Gel protectants like Zilactin and Orabase create a film "bandage" over the sore. (Some gels contain a numbing agent like benzocaine to temporarily block pain.) Avoid toothache medicines, however, especially if they contain the numbing agent eugenol. These products may actually irritate the canker sore and delay healing, says Michael A. Siegel, D.D.S., associate professor in the Department of Oral Medicine at the Dental School at the University of Maryland in Baltimore.

Swish cankers away. According to one study, antimicrobial mouth rinses like Listerine cut the pain of canker sores and accelerate the healing process, "perhaps by reducing the amount of bacteria in the mouth," says Dr. Rooney.

Suck on a lozenge. Medicated lozenges like Cepacol or Chloraseptic can help numb canker pain. (If you're in too much misery to eat, choose a lozenge with a stronger numbing agent like Xylocaine.)

Don't overdo the lozenges, though. "If your mouth is too numb, you might have trouble figuring out where the food is and accidentally bite your cheek!" says Dr. Rooney.

Prescription-Only Canker Cures

If over-the-counter remedies don't heal your canker sore, ask your doctor about these by-prescription-only treatments.

An Rx-strength gel. Your doctor may prescribe a gel like Orabase that contains the anti-inflammatory steroid Kenalog.

Medicated mouth rinse. For a serious outbreak, your doctor might prescribe a mouth rinse containing the antibiotic tetracycline. But *never* use this treatment if you're pregnant or think you might be: Tetracycline can permanently stain an unborn child's teeth.

Oral drugs for severe outbreaks. The oral steroid prednisone, which reduces inflammation, works very well on canker sores, says Dr. Siegel. But because of its side effects, prednisone is usually prescribed in high doses for a short time, which is safer than taking the drug for a longer duration.

Fever Blisters: Oral Enemy #1

Unlike canker sores, fever blisters usually appear on the outside of your mouth and along your lips. But you can also get them on your gums and the roof of your mouth, on your chin or cheeks—even in your nose. Unlike canker sores, which are round or oval and usually appear one at a time, cold sores are irregularly shaped and occur in crops of tiny blisters.

Fever blisters are caused by the herpes simplex virus. These blisters are also contagious, spread mostly by sharing eating utensils or drinking glasses or—unhappily—kissing. But romance rarely has anything to do with getting a cold sore. "We're usually already exposed to the type-one virus early in life," explains Dr. Rooney.

But what activates the virus and the cold sore in the first place? As with canker sores, experts suspect stress, the menstrual cycle and trauma to the mouth. You might also find you're more susceptible when you're run-down or when you have a cold or the flu. But the only well-documented culprit is the sun.

On-the-Spot Healing Hints

If you've temporarily shelved your lipstick as much to downplay the bubble on the edge of your lip as to ease its sting, soothe your cold sore with these quick remedies—and pick up a few tips on how to cope with the dratted blisters themselves.

Ice the cold sore site. As soon as you feel that telltale tingling, ice the spot to lower your skin's metabolic rate. "The virus can't turn over as fast, and this seems to minimize flare-ups for some people," says Dr. Siegel.

Bathe the blister. Some people dry up their blister by swabbing it before it pops with rubbing alcohol or 3 percent hydrogen peroxide. Don't wince—rubbing alcohol won't sting if the blister's still intact.

Bag your blister with tea. Cover the blister with a wet, cool tea bag. "The tannic acid and theobromine (a cousin of caffeine) in tea leaves can reduce a cold sore's inflammation," says Dr. Siegel.

Soothe sores with salve. Over-the-counter medicated salves and ointments like Blistex, Carmex and Campho-Phenique may ease the pain of fever blisters, although there's no proof they help heal them.

Don't apply a medicated product by touching the end of the tube to the sore itself; you can contaminate the product's contents, thereby reinfecting yourself with each use. Apply your salve or ointment with a cotton swab instead.

Don't use steroids on cold sores. Never use a canker treatment—namely, a prescription gel containing Kenalog—on a fever blister. "Hydrocortisone cream may help a canker sore, but if you use it on a fever blister, the steroid will cause it to spread," says Dr. Siegel.

Keep your blisters to yourself. "Fever blisters are most contagious while they're filled with fluid, but you can still infect someone until they're fully healed," says Dr. Siegel. Until then, kissing is out (especially kissing infants), and don't share glasses, silverware or straws. "Also, clean all your glasses and silverware thoroughly every time you use them," says Dr. Siegel.

Keep your hands off. Keep blisters clean and dry, but don't touch them: You may infect other parts of your body, including your eyes.

Keep the makeup away. Don't attempt to camouflage cold sores with cosmetics or concealers. "Applying and removing cover-ups may make things worse," says Dr. Siegel.

A Drug That Fights Ferocious Fever Blisters

If you're plagued by outbreak after outbreak of fever blisters, you may want to ask your doctor about whether the oral drug acyclovir (Zovirax), used to treat genital herpes, may also help reduce your fever blister flare-ups. The manufacturer of acyclovir, Burroughs-Wellcome, hasn't asked the Food and Drug Administration to review the drug's use for fever blisters. But some doctors prescribe it for that purpose.

In one multicenter study, researchers found that acyclovir prevented some outbreaks if it was taken before the blisters appeared. But some of the same researchers found that taking the drug after the blisters erupted didn't seem to help.

On the other hand, continuous daily therapy with oral acyclovir has reduced the frequency and severity of recurrences for people who suffer bouts of fever blisters as often as once a month.

CHAPTER SEVEN

Cellulite

Tactics against Cottage-Cheese Thighs

*I*t rolls around every year: bathing suit season. And it can be a long, hot summer if you spend it trying to camouflage the rippled, bumpy fat on your thighs, rear end or upper arms. But when you come right down to it, this dimpled fat—cellulite—is as unwelcome in January as it is in June.

Unhappily, there's no magic cream or lotion that can banish "cottage cheese" thighs. But don't fret: Cellulite may be forever, but it is possible to minimize its appearance. Here's how.

The Ripple Effect

In 1975 a best-selling book christened dimpled, orange-peel skin cellulite, giving a name to one of women's most maddening beauty problems. But most doctors agree: Cellulite isn't a special type of fat; it's just fat, period.

Cellulite's bulges and puckers appear when the connective fibers that anchor your skin to underlying muscle pull your skin inward, which pushes fat cells outward against your skin. (Think of the buttons on an overstuffed chair, which pull part of the chair's plushness tight while the rest plumps out.) Since women are genetically pro-

Cellulite "Remedies": What Works, What Won't

Many self-proclaimed beauty experts claim cellulite results from "toxins" trapped in your tissues and can be
eliminated by steering clear of caffeine, alcohol, cigarettes
and stress. Some beauty salon aestheticians even recommend treating cellulite by drawing these alleged "poisons"
from your body with a combination of massage and treatments formulated with flower, herb or plant extracts. But
these botanical treatments have never been scientifically
proven to work.

Neither have the many anticellulite gels, lotions and
creams on the market, including the very expensive potions
concocted with those plant and flower extracts or the new
thigh-shrinking creams that contain aminophylline (a drug
used to treat asthma). Some of the products temporarily
tighten and smooth the skin with ingredients that cause it
to swell for a few hours, sometimes a few days—but they
don't eliminate cellulite.

Also remember that anticellulite treatments are classified
as cosmetics, not drugs, and as such don't have to undergo
Food and Drug Administration testing or evaluation. So
you can try anticellulite body treatments or thigh creams if
you like, but don't expect them to melt away cellulite.

As for liposuction, it may be able to vacuum the stuffing
out of saddlebag thighs. But can it do anything for cellulite?
Perhaps.

Liposuction, the surgical method of suctioning fat from
the stomach, hips, thighs and other trouble spots, does get
rid of extra fat, and many woman are happy with the results. But the procedure can be unpredictable, says James J.
Leyden, M.D., professor of dermatology at the University
of Pennsylvania School of Medicine in Philadelphia. It's
impossible to know in advance whether liposuction will
result in uniformly smooth, undimpled skin. Face the facts:
The only way to battle cellulite—fat—is to burn it off with
diet and exercise.

grammed to store fat around their hips, thighs and behind, that's where most cellulite ends up.

Experts aren't sure why some of us dimple and others don't, or why some thin women get cellulite while other, heavier women remain ripple-free. "It's like asking why some of us have blue eyes or red hair—it's genetic," says Albert M. Kligman, M.D., Ph.D.

We do, however, know that men don't get cellulite because they tend to store fat around their middles rather than in the cellulite zone (thighs, hips and behind). Also, the skin's inner layer (the dermis), overlying the fat layer, is thicker in men, which helps hide dimples, and men's connective fibers are anchored differently. Lucky them!

Burn, Baby, Burn—Fat, That Is

While a cellulite-prone woman may never be completely cellulite-free, there is good news. If you shed fat, you'll most likely lose some of the lumps. So if you're battling cellulite, the first plan of attack is to exercise.

"Obviously, the less body fat you have, the less fat you have to store as cellulite," says James M. Swinehart, M.D., president of the Denver Dermatology Center. "Building up your muscle tone helps, too." While muscle weighs more than fat, it's also a lot more useful: The more muscle you have, the more calories you burn, even when you're at rest. "Muscle is the tissue that burns calories. Fat just sits around," explains Seattle nutritionist Susan M. Kleiner, R.D., Ph.D., author of *The High Performance Cookbook.*

By far, the most efficient way to burn fat and build muscle is by combining aerobic exercise with strength-training. It's a one-two punch: Aerobics, walking, jogging or swimming works off the fat and, presumably, some of the cellulite. Strength-training (doing leg lifts using ankle weights, for example, or working out on various weight-training machines) tones and builds your muscles. And cellulite or no cellulite, muscular areas like the hips, buttocks and thighs always look firmer and more youthful toned than untoned.

Fitness experts suggest you do aerobic exercise 30 minutes or more per session, three to five times a week. If you're new to exercise, get your doctor's okay first, and enlist a qualified instructor or personal trainer at a local gym or YMCA to make sure you're doing things correctly, for safety and maximum benefit.

Other Solutions for Orange-Peel Skin

Although there's no substitute for working up a good sweat, there are other methods you might try to minimize cellulite. Here's what the experts recommend.

Don't chew the fat. If you want to shed fat from your cellulite zone, shed it from your diet first by cutting back on rich desserts, crunchy fried snack foods, oily dressings and fatty meats.

Limit your fat intake to the recommended 20 to 30 percent of your daily calories, says Dr. Kleiner. "Calories from fat sources get stored as fat more readily than carbohydrate and protein calories," she notes. So nosh on more crunchy fruits and veggies, whole-grain breads and pasta, broiled chicken and low-fat yogurt.

If calculating percentage of calories from fat is too much bother, stick to a daily total intake of 40 to 50 grams of fat. Read labels for fat-gram content per serving, to help gauge, not guess, your intake.

Try massage. Some anticellulite products suggest you use them in tandem with massage. A cream makes massage easier, but it's the pounding, not the potions, that probably helps most, according to studies conducted by James J. Leyden, M.D., professor of dermatology at the University of Pennsylvania School of Medicine in Philadelphia, and his colleagues. "Massage won't get rid of your cellulite, but it's clearly helpful," says Dr. Leyden. "Massage breaks up fat cells, which makes it harder for fat to dimple."

Dr. Leyden suggests massaging trouble spots three times a day. "Massage takes dedication but costs you nothing to try," he says.

Rub in Retin-A. Retin-A (topical tretinoin), the derivative of vitamin A used to treat acne and wrinkles, may improve the appearance of cellulite when it's used in tandem with massage and exercise, says Dr. Kligman.

"When you use Retin-A, skin gets a bit thicker and firmer, and then the little fat pockets don't project through the skin as much," explains Dr. Kligman, who has studied Retin-A's effect on cellulite extensively.

But Retin-A isn't a miracle cure. "Cellulite is fat," notes Dr. Kligman. "You aren't going to improve it very much by putting creams on top of it."

Give yourself a break. If you've tried everything and still harbor a few unwanted ripples, don't fret. "You can be at your ideal weight and in great shape, yet still have dimples," says Dr. Leyden. His advice: Lighten up on yourself while you do what you can to trim down your puckers.

CHAPTER EIGHT

Chapped Lips

Handy Tips for Moister Lips

You can spend top dollar for lipstick, but if your lips are chapped and dry, even the most luscious lip color won't cover up the problem. Better to keep your lips smooth and moist before the damage is done.

Slicking on a good lip protectant (including moisturizing lipsticks) daily can keep your lips soft, smooth and kissable virtually year-round. But if your lips do crack, you can ease the pain, speed healing and put your lipstick back where it belongs—on your smoother, prettier lips. And while they'll probably pass on the lipstick, men can benefit from the tips in this chapter, too.

Lips Need Health Care of Their Own

Unlike your skin, your lips don't have oil glands to keep them lubricated and contain very little melanin, or pigment, to shield them from the sun. This lack of natural protection makes your lips extremely vulnerable to chapping—especially by the sun.

Like your skin, lips burn in both types of ultraviolet (UV) light that reach the Earth—ultraviolet-B (UVB), associated with sunburns and skin cancer, and ultraviolet-A (UVA), which can cause just as much skin damage over time. Even winter sun can brutalize your lips, particularly if you ski. "People don't associate skiing with sun exposure, but a tremendous amount of sun reflection bounces off snow," says Zoe Draelos, M.D., clinical assistant professor of dermatology at the Bowman Gray School of Medicine in Winston-Salem, North Carolina.

Along with the sun, cold winter weather (and its lip-chapping winds) and dry air take their toll on your lips. Home heating systems and air conditioners can leave indoor air—and lips—bone dry. Licking or biting your lips, getting a cold accompanied by a fever or taking certain over-the-counter and prescription medications can rough up your lips, too.

Three Ways to Chap-Proof Your Kisser

You can choose from three basic types of lip protection: plain lip balm, lip balms with added sunscreen and lip balms formulated with sunblock. While all of these products can keep lips smooth and pretty, you need to know how to use them—and when.

Lip balms. Formulated with emollients like petrolatum, lanolin, cocoa butter, aloe and sometimes wax, lip balms both prevent and heal chapped lips by sealing in moisture. Balms keep lips moist, not sun-safe. But used indoors, balms shield lips from dry indoor air and may even prevent cold-induced fever blisters. Chap Stick and Carmex are two good, basic lip balms.

Limit use of lip balm to an as-needed basis. Your lips could become overly dependent on it. "I've seen lip-balm junkies apply it eight times a day for years, and their lips eventually stop remoisturizing themselves," says Rodney S. W. Basler, M.D., head of a task force on sports medicine and assistant professor of dermatology at the University of Nebraska Medical Center in Omaha. So once your lips are healed, wean yourself off the balm.

Balms with added sunscreens. These products shield your lips from the sun and contain some of the same chemical sunscreens found in skin sunscreens, like padimate-O or oxybenzone. Most dermatologists recommend using a lip sunscreen with a sun protection factor, or SPF, of at least 15. Lip screens also protect your lips from other drying elements, like wind, salt water and chlorine, and may even keep you from sprouting a sun-induced fever blister.

Slick on a lip balm with sunscreen whenever you venture outdoors, be it to walk the dog, play tennis or bike through the park.

Apply the product 20 minutes before you go out to allow it to really sink in, and reapply after you swim, eat, drink or perspire.

To double your protection, choose a product that keeps lips moist and sun-safe, like the Body Shop's Honey Stick (with SPF 15) or Neutrogena Lip Moisturizer SPF 15, which is also PABA-free. (PABA, or para-aminobenzoic acid, is a chemical sunscreen that causes allergic reactions in some people.)

Balms with added sunblock. Physical sunblocks like zinc oxide and titanium dioxide protect your lips by diffusing and scattering all UV light. "Essentially, sunblocks have an infinite SPF," says Dr. Draelos. Best of all, physical sunblocks, which used to be available only as a gunky white paste, are now formulated to be invisible.

Choose a lip block (like Body Glove's Waterproof Sunblock Lip Balm SPF 25) if you'll be exposed to high doses of sun—while sailing or sunny-slope skiing, for example—and especially if you're prone to cold sores. "No one knows whether it's UVA or UVB that reactivates cold sores, so zinc oxide provides more complete protection from both," says Dr. Draelos.

To Zap Chapping, Keep Your Lips Sealed

A second or two of protective action practically ensures soft, smooth lips. So keep your lips chap-free by following these simple tips.

Reach for plain old petroleum jelly. To keep your lips moist and smooth, Albert M. Kligman, M.D., Ph.D., is a firm believer in unadorned, unmedicated petroleum jelly. Smooth on a dab up to four times a day to keep lips soft and supple.

Nourish lips nocturnally. Lips can dry out during the night, especially if you breathe through your mouth while you sleep or if the air in your bedroom is warm and dry. "It's a good idea to use lip balm at night even if you don't have chapped lips to prevent you from getting them," says Diana Bihova, M.D., clinical assistant professor of dermatology at New York University Medical Center in New York City.

Tote your lip protection. As we mentioned, use a lip balm with added sunscreens whenever you're outdoors. Tuck the product into your pocket or purse and take it everywhere.

Look out for lip-drying drugs. Prescription and over-the-counter drugs that work by drying out your skin or other tissues can have an unpleasant side effect: They can dry out your lips, too. So if you're taking Accutane (isotretinoin) for acne, decongestants, antihistamines or cold and cough products that dry out mucous membranes, diuretics or anticholinergics (antiperspiration drugs), load your lips with lip balm.

Also, keep drying skin-care products formulated with alcohol or benzoyl peroxide, such as astringents or blemish creams, off your lips.

Protect while You Primp

Keeping your lips smooth, soft and chap-free can be as simple as slicking on your favorite lipstick, says Albert M. Kligman, M.D., Ph.D. "Lipstick protects your lips. In fact, men have more cases of photodamaged lips than women."

For maximum protection, try moisturizing formulas like L'Oreal's Colour Riche Hydrating Lipcolour, Clinique's Remoisturizing Lipstick, Estee Lauder's Perfect or lipsticks with added sunscreen (lots of cosmetics companies, including Almay, Maybelline and Cover Girl, offer them). If you use regular lipstick, apply a plain balm or lip sunscreen underneath to further protect your lips.

Avoid matte (nonshiny) or mood lipsticks (the kind that are green or orange in the tube, but change color when you apply them) if your lips chap easily. These lipsticks can stain and dry lips, leaving them open to chapping or an allergic or irritant reaction. Go for the glossy instead.

If your lips are already a little dry, prep them for lip color with this easy treatment: Five minutes before you apply lipstick, smooth petroleum jelly over your lips. Then blot off the excess with a tissue. By the time you're ready to apply lip color, your lips will be softer and smoother. Explains Diana Bihova, M.D., clinical assistant professor of dermatology at New York University Medical Center in New York City, "Petroleum jelly fills in the cracks and creates a film on the surface of your lips. You can even put it over your lipstick."

If Your Lips Are Already Chapped . . .

You can't crack a smile with dry, cracked lips—but you don't have to grin and bear them, either. Ease the pain with these soothing tips.

Whip up a cure. For severely chapped lips, try Dr. Basler's favorite chapped lips recipe: Blend equal amounts of 1 percent hydrocortisone cream and Carmex and apply to painfully dry lips. "This works wonderfully on even the worst cases of chapped lips," he says.

Get off the stick. A waxy stick balm can drag painfully along already chapped lips. Try a softer, oilier squeeze- or roll-on formula, like Vaseline Intensive Care lip treatment, available in small tubes.

Use medicated balms cautiously. Dr. Kligman cautions against using medicated lip products, especially if they contain menthol. They may cause an allergic reaction in some people, says Dr. Basler. And some people may notice that their lips feel even drier after using a medicated balm. If this happens to you, "switch to a straight emollient, like petroleum jelly," advises Dr. Kligman.

Licking Lip-Chapping Habits

Licking and biting your lips can cause them to crack, dry out, even shred. Why give the sun, wind and cold more ammunition? Here's how to stop self-induced lip abuse.

Mind your tongue. Chances are, you're licking your lips unconsciously, says Dr. Bihova.

To break your habit, coat your lips with a flavor you just can't stand, suggests Dr. Draelos. "For instance, if you don't like anise, rub a licorice candy over your lips," she says.

Slather your lips with balm, too, suggests Dr. Basler. "It's logical to want to lick chapped lips, because the moisture soothes the second it hits your lips," he says. "So the best thing to do is to keep your lips moisturized." If you can find a balm in a flavor you don't like, you may be able to kill two birds with one stone.

Nix lip nipping. Biting chapped lips is adding insult to injury: Chewing away their protective mucous membrane can make them swollen and painful and may even lead to infection.

Keeping your lips well-coated with balm can help you quit your lip nipping. "If your lips are well-moisturized, the dead skin won't peel off as easily," says Dr. Basler. You can also try chewing on gum or celery rather than on your lips.

CHAPTER NINE

Dandruff and Related Problems

The Right Stuff for the White Stuff

Tired of constantly looking over your shoulder for those telltale flakes and wearing white, the only color sure to keep them from showing? Or is your scalp so scaly you're beginning to wonder whether you're part fish?

Dandruff isn't a serious medical problem, but it sure is a nuisance—and sometimes tricky to treat. Why? Because not all scalp flaking is simple dandruff, and *dandruff* is actually a catch-all term used to describe a number of scalp conditions.

If this news has you scratching your head in confusion (or just because your scalp's itching like crazy), you'll want to find out whether you have common dandruff or a peskier skin condition called seborrheic dermatitis, or seb derm. Then you can take steps to shake your case of flakes, or at least keep it under control.

The Flack over Flakes

To differentiate ordinary dandruff from the more stubborn and troublesome seb derm, check your scalp for the presence or absence of inflammation and oil. If you have dandruff, your scalp is probably dry, not oily, and shedding cells faster than normal, according to R. Jeffrey Herten, M.D., assistant clinical professor of dermatology at the University of California School of Medicine in Irvine.

"Normally, your skin cells fall off in microscopic amounts you can't see," says Dr. Herten. "But if the cells aren't shedding properly, or when your scalp is excessively dry, the cells form clusters and shed, which you see as little white specks. That's dandruff."

Seborrheic dermatitis is actually severe dandruff. Seb derm tends to be inflamed, with red or yellow scaly patches rather than dry flakes. Says Diana Bihova, M.D., clinical assistant professor of dermatology at New York University Medical Center in New York City, "You can have a scaliness all over your scalp or, in severe cases, an accumulation of crust. Some people's scalps get so itchy they'll scratch to the point of developing sores." What's more, seborrheic dermatitis can creep to oil-prone areas beyond your scalp: to your forehead, the nape of your neck, your eyebrows and eyelids, behind your ears and even the corners of your nostrils.

Most dermatologists agree that seborrheic dermatitis is caused by a naturally occurring yeast that lives on the surface and tips of your hair follicles and feeds on the oil on your scalp. An excess of this yeast incites dandruff and seborrheic dermatitis.

Seborrheic dermatitis tends to be a chronic condition. "It's something you learn to control and deal with," says Dr. Herten. Fortunately, most people generally get a yearly reprieve. Seborrheic dermatitis and dandruff tend to clear up in the summertime for reasons that are not completely understood.

But if your stress level builds up, so may your flakes. Emotional stress can trigger both seb derm and dandruff. "Stress has a significant role in the formation of dandruff," says Philip Kingsley, a British hair specialist with treatment centers in London and New York and author of *The Complete Hair Book*. "If you're prone to dandruff, it certainly does fluctuate with stress. And the more stress you're under, generally speaking, the worse it gets." Adds Dr. Bihova, "Even positive stress—landing a new job, buying a new home, getting married—is a common culprit."

So while you can't always control what life throws your way, trying to keep tranquil may help keep flakes off your shoulders.

Wash Those Flakes Right Out of Your Hair

Manufacturers have sought to fill your need for a flake-free scalp by formulating shampoo with various antidandruff ingredients not

A Case of Mistaken Identity

You just colored your hair. A few days later, you notice a lot of white collecting on your shoulders. How did you get that dandruff?

It may not be dandruff at all. Irritant or allergic contact dermatitis, a flaky, itchy skin condition that can be triggered by the chemicals in certain hair products, can look much like dandruff or seborrheic dermatitis.

Paraphenylenediamine, the ingredient in hair dyes, is a prime culprit, which is why you should always perform a patch test before you color. The chemicals used to straighten and perm hair can irritate your scalp, too, even if they're only on your scalp a short time.

If your scalp flakes or becomes red or inflamed after you perm, color or straighten your hair, consult a dermatologist to find out whether you have contact dermatitis and, if so, how you can treat it.

found in regular shampoos. But which shampoo you choose depends on whether you're battling dandruff or seborrheic dermatitis.

If you have dandruff, pick a shampoo formulated with selenium sulfide (Selsun Blue), sulfur (MG217 Medicated Tar-Free) or zinc pyrithione (Zincon). If you have seborrheic dermatitis, try a shampoo formulated with coal tar (Tegrin) or salicylic acid (P & S shampoo)—they're stronger. All of these ingredients work by reducing the scaling caused by the excess yeast.

Be prepared to keep switching dandruff shampoos, says Dr. Bihova. You might find that your favorite brand eventually stops working as your scalp builds up a tolerance to the key ingredient.

Be Tough on Flakes, Tender on Your Hair

When it comes to keeping the snow off your shoulders, medicated shampoos can be extremeley effective. But they do have a drawback: The harder these shampoos work on your scalp, the harder they can be on your hair, especially chemically processed hair.

"Think of the hair cuticle as a raincoat around each strand of your hair," says Dr. Herten. "When you wash your hair with those strong shampoos, you really destroy the cuticle." Without its protective raincoat, your hair absorbs and then loses water more rapidly, ultimately becoming brittle and unmanageable.

Before you opt for a medicated shampoo, try washing your hair every day with a regular shampoo, suggests Kingsley. Or use a medicated shampoo only every third or fourth day, sudsing with a mild product on the days in between, says Dr. Herten.

You might also try one of the dandruff shampoos with added conditioners, like Selsun Gold for Women or Head & Shoulders. "Conditioners also coat the scalp, which is one of the reasons they cut down on scaliness," explains Dr. Herten. Some companies make both a medicated shampoo and conditioner. Try, for example, Neutrogena's coal-tar-based T/Gel Conditioner, meant to be used after washing with T/Gel or T/Sal shampoo, which is formulated with salicylic acid.

Pick a medicated shampoo even more carefully if you have colored or permed hair, says Dr. Herten. For example, coal tar can darken gray, blonde or color-treated hair.

If you're considering coloring or perming your hair, wait until your dandruff or seb derm clears up so you won't hit your hair with the double whammy of chemical processing and dandruff shampoos.

More Ways to Scale Down

Lathering up with a medicated shampoo isn't the only way to defeat dandruff or seb derm. Give these remedies a try, too.

Sprinkle your scalp with mouthwash. An antibacterial mouthwash like Listerine is an effective home treatment for dandruff because it keeps the yeast level under control, says Kingsley. "Cut the mouthwash with 50 percent distilled water, sprinkle it on your scalp after you shampoo and rub it in," he advises. "If you keep the bacteria under control, the chances of getting dandruff are very much less." In fact, he suggests this treatment before you even try a dandruff shampoo. If you think the smell of mouthwash may bother you (or other people), try this treatment well before you go to work or a social engagement to give the odor time to dissipate.

Scale down between shampoos. Try an over-the-counter scalp-treatment product to help calm inflammation and irritation between shampoos. A 1 percent hydrocortisone solution, like Scalpicin or Cortizone-10 Scalp Itch Formula Liquid, is even better. "It's easier to massage into your scalp than a cream and is invisible and non-greasy," says Dr. Bihova.

But these products aren't long-term remedies. "Hydrocortisone won't get rid of yeast or control oil production," says Dr. Herten. Adds Dr. Bihova, "The long-term use of even something mild enough to be sold over the counter can cause problems. Any cortisone, hydrocortisone or steroid preparation, no matter how weak it is, can lead to side effects like thinning of the skin and broken blood vessels."

Hydrocortisone also tends to be less effective over time, and using it too often may make your seb derm worse. So use this product only when you have redness, not as a preventive measure.

"Also, if you use a hydrocortisone product on flaky eyebrows, be especially careful to keep it away from your eyes," says Dr. Bihova.

Prescription Shampoos to the Rescue

Generally, over-the-counter products are for mild or occasional dandruff or seb derm; they don't always work on stubborn or persistent cases. You may need to see a dermatologist, who can prescribe stronger treatments and identify which works best for you.

To control severe dandruff, Dr. Bihova prescribes Selsun Rx, which contains roughly double the concentration of the active ingredient, selenium sulfide, than the company's over-the-counter product Selsun Blue.

For severe cases of seborrheic dermatitis, Dr. Bihova and many other dermatologists prescribe Nizoral, an antifungal shampoo. Its key ingredient, ketoconazole, attacks the yeast problem directly.

What's more, ketoconazole is milder than selenium sulfide. In a Canadian study of 246 people, dermatologists pitted a selenium sulfide–based dandruff shampoo against one formulated with ketoconazole. Both shampoos worked as well on flakes, but the ketoconazole didn't cause the side effects that the group using the selenium sulfide product experienced—itching, burning, skin rashes and staining of the hair.

"Also, Nizoral doesn't do a lot of damage to hair—the shampoo itself isn't harsh," says Dr. Herten. "It's costly, but it's a real breakthrough for a lot of people."

CHAPTER TEN

Eczema

Soothing the Itch You Just Can't Scratch

*E*ver had an itchy, scaly rash on your finger that faded when you stopped wearing a new ring? Or caught poison ivy when you stumbled onto a previously uncharted patch of underbrush while walking your dog?

Eczema, or dermatitis, as it's also called, covers an entire range of red, itchy, scaly skin irritations. Some types of eczema are temporary, like poison ivy. Other types, like atopic dermatitis (AD), are more persistent.

But whether your eczema's caused by a run-in with a poison plant or a chronic skin condition like AD, you can ease the itch and—in many cases—clear your skin with quick, easy remedies. Even better, you can minimize AD flare-ups by taking simple preventive measures and speed healing with by-prescription-only relief.

ID'ing the Itch

"All the eczemas tend to overlap," says Jon M. Hanifin, M.D., professor of dermatology at Oregon Health Sciences University in Portland and an eczema expert. "If you have one type of dermatitis, your skin is going to be more sensitive to others."

The three most common types of eczema are AD, contact derma-

titis and nummular dermatitis. While they all share the same sur-
name, it's virtually the only thing these skin conditions have in
common.

Atopic dermatitis. AD, the most common and most severe form of
eczema, is hereditary; the first flare-up often occurs in early child-
hood. People who have it (or their family members) often suffer from
hay fever or asthma as well. Having AD also makes you more susceptible to other types of eczema, like hand and eyelid dermatitis.

The skin of people who have atopic dermatitis doesn't hold water,
making it dry, scaly and itchy. "Dry skin is an almost constant feature
of AD," says Albert M. Kligman, M.D., Ph.D. "AD starts in infancy
as red patches on the face and forearms. But in adults, dry skin may
be the only sign of it." During flare-ups, however, scratching the skin
or infections can cause crusted sores to develop.

Almost anything can trigger a flare-up of AD, including stress, cold
weather and low humidity, heat and high humidity or a mild staph or
bacterial infection on the surface of your skin. Even a common cold
can cause AD to flare. So if you have this condition, Dr. Hanifin recommends you see a doctor to treat any infection immediately.

Contact dermatitis. There are actually two types of contact dermatitis. Irritant contact dermatitis (ICD) is caused by direct contact
with a substance even nonallergic people may react to, including
soaps, astringents and other skin-care products that contain alcohol,
cosmetics and perfumes and harsh household detergents.

ICD is characterized by red, tight skin that may crack or blister.
"There are literally thousands of irritants," says Dr. Kligman. "Stronger ones like kerosene or gasoline will irritate your skin on the
first exposure, while weaker ones like soaps injure your skin less
readily."

So how do you know what's riling your skin? If the rash is on your
hands, suspect a case of ICD. Then take a close look at what you're
handling at work. So-called hand dermatitis often crops up on the
job. "Getting your hands into soap and water or cleaning solutions
can make them crack and dry out," says Dr. Hanifin. "That's basically what ICD is—cracking, drying out and tightness."

By contrast, allergic contact dermatitis (ACD) doesn't irritate your
skin. It's an allergic response triggered by your immune system, the
body's first line of defense against disease and infection. Nickel-
plated jewelry, preservatives and fragrances are a few common allergens. So are poison oak, ivy and sumac. Yet not everyone is

allergic to these plants. Some people react after handling clothing that's been exposed, while others can roll in the stuff without harm.

A flare-up of ACD begins with redness, swelling and a breakout of itchy blisters, often arranged in a telltale pattern: in lines if a poison plant touched your skin or in a circle if the offender was a nickel-plated earring or ring. Unless you know exactly what caused the reaction, you may want to have a patch test, in which common allergens are applied to the skin. The test can often sleuth a suspected allergen so you can prevent another outbreak.

ICD is more common than ACD. But it can be harder to identify its cause.

Nummular dermatitis. This rash appears in red, scaly, circular patches that may also weep or bleed. Nummular dermatitis is difficult to treat because "no one knows what causes it," says Dr. Hanifin.

Is It Something You Ate?

Your skin seems to get riled every time you pop a peanut into your mouth or dunk your Oreo into a glass of milk. Is it your imagination? No. Food allergies play a significant role in eczema flare-ups, says Jon M. Hanifin, M.D., professor of dermatology at Oregon Health Sciences University in Portland and an eczema expert. What's more, just touching—let alone eating—the food can do a number on your skin.

Most dermatologists agree that the six worst eczema-triggering foods—also called the big six—are:

→ Eggs
→ Milk
→ Peanuts
→ Wheat
→ Soy
→ Seafood

Call your doctor if you experience an allergic reaction after eating any of these foods.

"It just has to be treated symptomatically." People over 60 with nummular dermatitis, however, often have a history of dry, scaly skin, especially in winter, adds Dr. Kligman.

High-Speed Help for a Sudden Rash

If you're pretty sure that what you have is an outright allergy rather than nonallergic eczema or dermatitis, taking these steps can spell fast relief.

Wash off quick. If you've frolicked in a bed of poison oak, ivy or sumac, rinse off as soon as possible. "Jump in a river if you have to!" says Dr. Hanifin. When you get home, wash your clothing and anything else that might have been contaminated, "from your dog to your Frisbee," he adds.

Bathe in oatmeal. Soak in a bath to which you've added about two cups of a colloidal (finely ground) oatmeal bath product like Aveeno. Or tie up the same amount of real oatmeal in an old nylon stocking and toss it into your tub.

Dry up the itch. Calamine lotion may reduce the itching of ACD and cool down your skin and help dry up the rash.

Treat a rash coldly. Cool compresses can relieve the itching. "Apply them the minute the itching starts and use them for as long as you need to," says Dr. Hanifin.

Don't get sensitive. Don't use anti-itch products that contain local anesthetics. "All the 'caines' like benzocaine are very strong allergens, and you run the risk of developing another contact dermatitis," Dr. Hanifin explains.

Heal with hydrocortisone. An over-the-counter 1 percent hydrocortisone cream or ointment can reduce itching and inflammation. Alexander A. Fisher, M.D., clinical professor of dermatology at New York University Medical Center in New York City prefers ointments because they usually contain few or no skin-irritating preservatives. "Spread on a thin film of the cream, ideally after baths or cool compresses, two or three times a day," says Dr. Hanifin.

If all else fails, ask about prednisone. In the past, doctors tended to treat severe allergic reactions that continue to spread—poison oak, for example—with the oral steroid prednisone. But that's changing, says Dr. Hanifin. "We're finding that some of the very high potency steroid creams will stop the blisters from spreading and save you from having to take prednisone." But an allergic reaction can sometimes be so ferocious at the onset that prednisone is the only treatment that helps, he adds.

Eight Great Ways to Soothe Eczema

If you're itching for relief from AD or ICD, these treatments can curb your urge to scratch. This is important, because the less you scratch, the less chance of infection—and the quicker your skin will heal.

The oatmeal soak. As with ACD, soaking in a bath to which you've added an oatmeal product like Aveeno may reduce the itching and irritation.

Moisturize, moisturize, moisturize. "Some people seem to outgrow AD because they learn to moisturize properly, which prevents their skin from cracking and irritants from entering the cracks," says Dr. Hanifin.

But not just any thin, drippy lotion will do. "Lotions are the enemy," says Dr. Hanifin. "They just dry you out—there's very little oil in them. You have to use an oil-rich moisturizer that doesn't pour—that is, something solid, like Nivea or Aquaphor. You can also use the 'gold standard' of emollients—petroleum jelly."

Avoid any moisturizer formulated with fragrances or preservatives, especially if you have ICD, says Dr. Fisher. "Apply the moisturizer to a small portion of your skin first to see if your skin reacts."

Come clean without causing a rash. "AD's most significant trigger factor is failing to seal in your skin's absorbed moisture after you bathe or shower," says Dr. Hanifin. Irritant reactions can cause extremely dry skin as well. So moisturize within three minutes of stepping out of the tub or after washing your hands if you have hand eczema. If you swim, grease up after your laps, too.

Fight the itch with ice. Apply a plastic bag of ice cubes or crushed ice to itchy, inflamed skin. "Ice is the best thing you can use to fight the urge to scratch," says Rodney S. W. Basler, M.D., head of a task force on sports medicine and assistant professor of dermatology at the University of Nebraska Medical Center in Omaha. Says Dr. Fisher, "It's especially good for cutting the swelling or redness of ICD." Applying cool compresses is another soothing option.

Wear natural fabrics and loose clothing. Don natural fabrics that "breathe," like cotton. They let air circulate around your skin, keeping it dry and comfortable. Avoid synthetic fabrics and wool. (While wool is a natural fabric, its scratchiness can irritate your skin.) And don't wear anything that makes you perspire: To keep cool, layer your clothing, suggests Dr. Hanifin.

Don't sweat it. Avoid strenuous exercise during flare-ups of AD or a bout with ICD: Perspiring can irritate your skin. Also, wear light sleepwear and turn down the thermostat at night so you won't perspire while you sleep.

A rash decision: hydrocortisone. According to Dr. Hanifin, "People with eczema should use a steroid cream any time their skin starts to redden or itch." As with ACD, a drugstore 1 percent hydrocortisone cream should be enough to calm the itching, although your doctor can prescribe stronger versions.

But don't overuse hydrocortisone cream. "It's a wonderful treatment," says Dr. Hanifin, but long-term use can cause side effects like thinning of the skin and stretch marks. Also avoid using it around your eyes. Dr. Hanifin suggests using the cream for a few days at the onset of redness, "then trying to get by with just your moisturizer." You can also boost a hydrocortisone cream's effectiveness by topping it with your moisturizer, says Dr. Basler.

Try antihistamines. Experts disagree on whether antihistamines (drugs used to relieve allergy symptoms) really help relieve the itch of eczema. But you may want to try them to see if they work for you. Dr. Kligman says newer antihistamines like Tavist, Benadryl and Chlor-Trimeton "won't make you sleepy and may block the action of histamine, the chemical that causes the itching."

If Your Eczema Gets Out of Hand . . .

If you can't get relief on your own, a doctor may be able to help you control your eczema with these treatments.

Rx-strength steroid creams. Prescription-strength steroid creams, like Cuteivate, Topicort, Westcort and Lidex (triamcinolone), can soothe eczema's itching and inflammation. But like their over-the-counter counterparts, these stronger products can cause thinning of the skin and stretch marks. "It's a constant fight to use just enough of these steroid creams to keep the symptoms under control," says Dr. Hanifin.

Soak up some "sun." Phototherapy with ultraviolet-B (UVB) lamps and doctor-monitored sun exposure often improves chronic AD. Undergoing phototherapy has its risks—skin cancer and premature aging of the skin. But experts say this therapy's benefits outweigh its risks.

Don't try these treatments on your own. Phototherapy can make the skin extremely sensitive to sunlight. And psoralens, the drugs that are used in a form of phototherapy called PUVA (psoralens and ultraviolet-A) make skin photosensitive for 24 hours after treatment. If you opt for either UVB or PUVA treatments, it's wise to avoid the sun altogether or slather a strong sunscreen over every inch of bare flesh. And talk to your doctor about protecting yourself from a sunburnlike reaction, advises Dr. Hanifin.

Clear up the mystery itch. If using steroid creams and moisturizing diligently do not improve your eczema, you may have ACD, says Dr. Hanifin. (He once treated four eczema patients who turned out to be allergic to their steroid creams.) The only way to find out once and for all whether your eczema is caused by allergens is to get a patch test. There are numerous allergens that may be causing your rash—substances you work with, including latex (natural rubber) gloves, food you've eaten or touched (in the case of hand dermatitis) and dust mites, grasses and animal dander.

The last resort. Because prescription drugs used to treat eczema can cause serious side effects, they're often the remedy of last resort. Prednisone can cause brittle bones and cataracts. Cyclosporine, used to treat psoriasis as well as AD, can lead to kidney problems, and eczema usually flares up when you go off the drug, says Dr. Hanifin.

Researchers are working to find new drugs that treat eczema without the damaging side effects. Gamma interferon, a natural body product that reduces the body's inflammatory responses, "may lessen AD's severity and provide the best hope for the future," says Dr. Hanifin.

See also the chapter on dandruff and related problems (chapter 9).

CHAPTER ELEVEN

Hives

Welcome Relief for Troubled Skin

The owner of a small but well-known cosmetics company once told me that the most stressful time in her life was when she had hives for three years straight. Being in the beauty business, she had access to the top doctors in New York. But not one could figure out what was triggering her breakouts: Her hives would erupt without warning and for no apparent reason, often right before an important meeting or a business trip. "It's hard to create a good impression with itchy welts all over your body, especially when you're trying to sell yourself as a skin-care expert!" she says.

Then one day her hives stopped as mysteriously as they had started. But hives often defy explanation.

There are two types of hives: chronic and acute. Chronic hives—the kind the cosmetics store owner had—have no identifiable cause, can last for days (sometimes weeks and months) and ebb and flare without warning. Acute hives appear suddenly, usually fade quickly and are most likely triggered by an allergic reaction to certain substances, especially foods.

The good news is, with acute hives, the first outbreak can be the last—it's simply a matter of avoiding the trigger. And while you can't control a flare-up of chronic hives, you can minimize its discomfort—and, even better, take steps to prevent recurrences.

The Buzz about Hives

About 20 percent of us will experience urticaria, or hives—itchy, swollen bumps—at least once in our lives. These harmless but annoying welts burst into bloom when certain cells release histamine, a chemical that creates the almost unbearable urge to itch. Your blood vessels dilate, leak fluid into the area and voilà—pop go the hives.

The bumps (doctors call them wheals) can be as tiny as a pea or as large as a plate and last from a few hours to a few days. Then, as if by magic, your body switches into reverse: The fluid is reabsorbed and blood vessels return to normal.

Compared to chronic hives, which can last up to six weeks or longer, most outbreaks of acute hives are sudden and short-lived. And acute hives can explode so fast you may know immediately what caused them. So if you think those strawberries are responsible for your misery, your doctor can give you a prick test to confirm whether your hives were brought on by an allergic reaction.

The Hives Hall of Blame

If acute hives are making you miserable and you're stumped as to their cause, consider these possible perpetrators.

Food. Shellfish, fish, peanuts, nuts, milk, eggs and wheat can all cause hives. But since food allergies affect only 2 percent of adults, and testing for diet-induced hives is expensive, think before you test. If you experience nausea, vomiting and diarrhea along with the hives every time you eat nuts, eggs or whatever, the problem is apt to be food-induced. If you have hives but no other symptoms, something else is to blame.

"If the hives are food-induced, the only 'treatment' is avoiding that food," says William O. Wagner, M.D., head of the Section of Allergy and Immunology in the Department of Pulmonary and Critical Care Medicine at the Cleveland Clinic Foundation.

Drugs. Penicillin and everyday aspirin are the most common culprits, but even an allergy shot can cause welts. Take a complete inventory of every drug you take over the course of a month, then ask your doctor if there's a way to eliminate the offender.

Infections. Hepatitis B and mononucleosis can cause hives, too, and so can thyroid and lupus-type diseases, although that's rare. "If you have symptoms that are worrying you, get a physical and some basic lab tests," says Jon M. Hanifin, M.D., professor of dermatology at Oregon Health Sciences University in Portland.

Chronic hives are hardly ever from an allergy, but whatever's causing them can keep them coming back for years. Worse, with chronic hives, all a prick test tells you is what isn't causing the problem.

Still, some persistent detective work can pay off. "Finding out what's causing the hives often depends on the enthusiasm of doctor and patient," says Dr. Hanifin.

If you can't discover what's triggering chronic hives, even partial answers are reassuring. Says Dr. Wagner, "While it can be frustrating that you still have the hives, finding out you're an otherwise healthy person should be helpful, because you won't have to go nuts about keeping food diaries or worrying about an underlying illness."

When It's Not Something You Ate

Hives aren't always caused by something you ate or drank. There are three other types: contact hives, physical hives and exercise-induced hives.

Contact hives are triggered by an allergy that causes hives to flare when a certain substance comes in contact with your skin, like cat dander. Handling certain raw foods can cause contact hives as well: For example, some people react after handling shellfish, although they have no problem eating it cooked. A prick test can reveal the

How to Handle Severe Hives

Although hives aren't usually life-threatening, severe cases can cause the throat to swell, cutting off breathing. Should you ever get hives in your throat or mouth, get help *immediately*. Then talk to your doctor about prescribing a medication called epinephrine to have ready for future emergencies.

You may also experience hives if you're allergic to latex. A wide variety of medical equipment, including catheters and hot-water bottles, are made of latex, so having a tube or nozzle inserted into your body could cause a potentially life-threatening reaction. So alert all doctors and health workers to your allergy, and carry this information in your wallet the way people allergic to penicillin do.

source of your allergy, and then you can simply avoid it.

Exposure to heat, cold, the sun, water or a hot environment like a hot tub can raise a feverish crop of physical hives (called physical urticaria). Even the pressure on your skin from a binding undergarment can cause this type of hives. Again, avoidance (and, in many cases, antihistamines) is the usual treatment for physical hives.

If you're prone to them, working up a sweat may trigger exercise-induced hives. This reaction is a rare response to the natural rise in body temperature that occurs with strenuous exercise like aerobics.

But exercise-induced hives are usually mild, and taking antihistamines (see below) may keep you from feeling itchy while you exercise. Also, try low- or no-sweat activities like walking, which make you less likely to perspire and cause a flare-up, says Dr. Wagner.

Antihive Strategies that Work

If, despite avoidance tactics, you still break out, try these emergency relief tips.

Don't scratch! Easier said than done, you say? Try wearing cotton gloves to keep your "trigger fingers" off your welts.

Calm hives with hydrocortisone—cautiously. If your hives are severe, you can soothe the itch with an over-the-counter hydrocortisone cream, says Karl R. Beutner, M.D., assistant clinical professor of dermatology at the University of California at San Francisco. But don't use it too long. "Avoid long-term use of hydrocortisone cream for hives, because hives can last for years," says Dr. Beutner. And if you use hydrocortisone for years, he says, you're virtually guaranteed side effects like thinning of the skin and stretch marks.

Carry antihistamines. Try taming your welts with an over-the-counter antihistamine. The most common treatment for hives, these drugs counteract the effects of histamine, help prevent new hives and curb the itch—which is crucial, because "hives can get bigger and itch even more if they're scratched," says Dr. Wagner.

If drugstore antihistamines don't help, your doctor may prescribe a nonsedating prescription antihistamine like Seldane, Hismanal or Claritin or a combination of antihistamines, including Zantac.

Heal hives with tranquillity. Stress can aggravate chronic hives. So try not to worry about them, says Dr. Wagner. "If you can suppress the hives entirely for a couple of weeks, quite often you'll break the cycle," he says.

CHAPTER TWELVE

Large Pores

Treatments for Skin That's the Pits

*I*nvisible pores have been touted as a hallmark of beautiful skin. Yet more than a few of us look in the mirror and confront a complexion whose texture looks more like the surface of the moon than satin-smooth. Maybe we should all stop peering into our magnifying mirrors!

Unfortunately, it's impossible to actually shrink your pores. But you can take steps to avoid making pores even larger and learn makeup techniques that will make them less noticeable.

When Pores Grow Wrong

Pores are tiny openings in the skin—the points of entry of hair follicles, sweat glands and oil glands, from which oil flows to the surface of your skin.

If you're bemoaning your large pores, don't! They serve a purpose: to secrete oil. The size of the oil glands located on your nose, cheeks and chin determines the size of your pores in these areas. In fact, if your pores weren't the size they are, you'd likely end up with a bigger problem: pimples. "Too much oil trying to drain from too-tiny pores could lead to blemishes," says Amy Newburger, M.D., associate clinical professor of dermatology at the College of Physicians and Surgeons of Columbia University and assistant attending physician at Presbyterian Hospital in New York City.

To prevent pores from enlarging in the first place, don't squeeze blackheads: It can rupture the hair follicle, causing scarring that permanently enlarges that pore, explains Dr. Newburger.

Also, stay out of the sun. As you get older, the damaging effects of the sun on your skin will finally catch up with your pores. "Sun damage can cause blackheads, which enlarge the pores. Then, as your pores try to expand, the material in them gets trapped," says Melvin L. Elson, M.D., medical director of the Dermatology Center in Nashville and co-author of *The Good Look Book*. So if you haven't already begun to wear a strong sunscreen, now's the time to start.

In Search of Shrink-to-Fit Pores

Experts agree that you can't reduce the size of your pores. "Pore size is inherited, and there's no way you can get around that," explains Zoe Draelos, M.D., clinical assistant professor of dermatology at the Bowman Gray School of Medicine in Winston-Salem, North Carolina. But you can make pores look less noticeable. Here's how.

Keep your skin clean. "Blemishes will make your pores more visible, so keep your face clean," says Diana Bihova, M.D., clinical assistant professor of dermatology at New York University Medical Center in New York City.

That doesn't mean you should scrub with harsh cleansers; it may spur your skin to generate more oil, and the more oil your skin pumps out, the larger your pores can get. Cleanse gently with a mild soap instead.

By the way, you may have heard that you can "close" your pores by steaming your face or alternately turning the water in your shower hot and cold. But this is the beauty equivalent of an old wives' tale: Pores can't be opened and closed like a window!

Use an astringent—sparingly. Alcohol-based skin-care products, like Sea Breeze, can temporarily close pores by irritating the skin, creating a swelling effect around the pores. But don't use too much astringent, too often—you may close your pores but end up with dry, flaky skin. Better to save an astringent for special occasions—before a big night out, for example. The pore-tightening effect is temporary, however—an hour or so.

Mask the problem. Face masks—especially those formulated with clay—draw out some oil from your skin, which will temporarily make your pores appear smaller. But they can also dry out your skin if you're not careful. Choose a brand formulated specifically for your skin type (dry, oily or normal) and follow directions to the letter. If you have sensitive skin, you probably shouldn't use masks at all.

Apply any mask thickly—too thin an application can work too well, causing parched, tight skin.

Rx Cures for Too-Large Pores

If regular cleansing isn't enough to clear blocked pores, relief may be as close as your dermatologist. The following are the most common pore-minimizing procedures.

Try a facial. Dermatologist-performed facials, which can include the removal of blackheads, are another pore-declogging option. Though you shouldn't squeeze blackheads yourself, a dermatologist knows how to remove blackheads without damaging your skin.

Peel off the plugs. A light peel with glycolic acid—a very mild alpha hydroxy acid (AHA) and an extremely popular beauty treatment—may also purge plugged pores, making them look slightly smaller. To be on the safe side, have the peel performed by a dermatologist.

Reach for Retin-A. Available by prescription only, Retin-A (topical tretinoin)—a derivative of vitamin A used to treat wrinkles and acne—can remove blackheads that are clogging your pores, which will minimize their appearance to some degree, says Dr. Bihova. A Retin-A regimen can also help shrink pores enlarged by sun exposure.

A Pore-Perfecting Makeup Plan

If you can't beat 'em, hide 'em—your pores, that is. And the right makeup can work wonders, hiding large pores and creating an illusion of smooth texture. "The only reason you can see pores is because they cast a shadow," says Dr. Newburger. "If you use a dewy or semidewy makeup that reflects light evenly, your pores will be more visible. A nonshiny, powdery makeup reflects light unevenly, so you won't see the pores as well."

These skin-care and makeup tips from Laura Geller, makeup artist and owner of Laura Geller Make-Up Studios, a cosmetics store in New York City, can help minimize the appearance of large pores.

Moisturizer: Water-based is best. "If you need to moisturize, use a water-based product," says Geller. "If you use one that's too oily, your foundation won't stay as matte as it could." Nivea Visage No Oil, All-Moisture Hydrogel is one of many you can try.

Foundation: Go to the matte. For a matte (nonshiny) look, Geller prefers a water-based liquid foundation. Check a foundation's label: Words like *water-based*, *oil-controlling* and *matte finish* will tip you off.

If you have mature skin and large pores, try a water-based cream foundation, which contains a small amount of oil. This type of cream formula fits the bill if you have large pores, says Geller, "because the base is still more water than oil."

You can also use a stick foundation (also called pan- or cream-stick foundation), whose very heavy coverage can cover pores completely. "These are oil-based, so you'll have to powder them down to remove the shine," says Geller. But because of its oil content, don't use a stick foundation if you have blemishes or breakout-prone skin.

Whichever foundation you use, apply it with a latex makeup sponge. If you're allergic to latex, use any smooth-surfaced sponge. "Using a sponge keeps the oil and bacteria on your fingers off your face, and foundation blends more smoothly and lasts longer," says Geller.

Powder: Use no-glow for pores. Choose a loose, talc-based flat (noniridescent) powder and apply it with a velour puff. "Applying powder with a brush only takes down the shine temporarily," says Geller. "But rolling the powder onto your skin with the velour puff sets the foundation and powder together and will keep your skin matte for as long as possible."

Blusher: Powder is best. A powdered blusher will cut shine even further. "If you prefer using cream rouge, apply it after your foundation, then set it with the loose powder," says Geller.

See also the chapter on sunscreen (chapter 28).

CHAPTER THIRTEEN

Psoriasis

Give Your Skin the All-Clear

Mention psoriasis and that old TV commercial catch-phrase "the heartbreak of psoriasis" comes to mind. The ad may have tickled the public's collective funny bone, but psoriasis is never a laughing matter if you're one of the four million people in the United States who live with this common skin disorder.

You may not realize how common, because psoriasis is so often hidden. But it might be easier to cover up the physical evidence of psoriasis—intense itching, unsightly scaling and occasional pain—than to conceal the emotional distress many people with psoriasis may feel because of the condition's appearance.

While there's not yet a cure for psoriasis, there's reason to be hopeful: Treatment is more effective than ever. But just as important, there's lots you can do to keep psoriasis from interfering with your looks—and your life.

Why Skin Cells Go Crazy

When you have psoriasis, your skin cells run amok. While it normally takes about 30 days for new cells to reach the surface of your skin, in psoriasis they surface in just 3 days—much too fast to be shed. These out-of-control skin cells form plaques—pink, raised patches covered by silvery white scales.

Experts aren't sure what causes psoriasis, but they do know it tends to run in families and most commonly hits in the teen years or middle age. Psoriasis tends to ebb and flare, although obesity, stress, smoking, certain drugs (Quinidine, a heart medication, and Inderal, a high blood pressure medication, to name two) or even a simple infection like a sore throat can aggravate outbreaks. Or you could go years without a flare-up; that's the nature of this chronic but very unpredictable condition.

Psoriasis can be mild or extremely severe. Fortunately, most people escape with a few small patches on their elbows, knees or scalp. About 90 percent of people with psoriasis will also develop thick, dented or pitted fingernails. And about 10 percent develop a form of arthritis associated with psoriasis that resembles rheumatoid arthritis.

Rx Mission: Remission

Having a doctor monitor your condition can make it easier for you to cope with psoriasis—emotionally as well as physically. "Everyone with severe psoriasis should get medical help," says Albert M. Kligman, M.D., Ph.D.

The three most common treatments for psoriasis are topical treatments (applied to the skin), light therapy (called phototherapy) and oral drugs. Topical treatments, including steroids, calcipotriene (a cream-based derivative of vitamin D) and anthralin, reduce scaling and inflammation. Phototherapy, or exposure to ultraviolet-B light, helps clear psoriasis, while another form of light therapy, PUVA (psoralens and ultraviolet-A light), reduces cell growth. Oral drugs like methotrexate and cyclosporine also inhibit cell growth and reduce inflammation.

The treatments that work best, however, may also cause serious side effects. Taken in excess, methotrexate may cause liver disease, while PUVA ups the risk of skin cancer and steroids can thin the skin and occasionally aggravate the psoriasis itself. Moreover, the effectiveness of these treatments tends to decrease over time as your skin builds up a resistance to them.

To lower the risks and heighten effectiveness, these treatments are often juggled or used in alternating combinations—a strategy called rotational therapy. "Psoriasis can go into remission with any of these treatments, but the goal is to find combination treatments that make the remissions last longer," says Alan Menter, M.D., clinical director of the National Psoriasis Tissue Bank at Baylor University Medical Center in Dallas and chairman of the dermatology department of that university. Currently under development are a vitamin A–based gel that eases psoriasis without the side effects of steroids and a topical version of methotrexate, which may be less risky, since less of the drug is absorbed through the skin.

Calcipotriene "seems to 'reset' psoriasis at a much less severe level, although it may not clear skin completely," says Nicholas J. Lowe, M.D., clinical professor of dermatology at the UCLA School of Medicine and director of the Skin Research Foundation of California in Santa Monica. "It's very safe, doesn't thin the skin like corticosteroids and can be used in tandem with light therapy." But calcipotriene can irritate skin, so Dr. Lowe doesn't recommend using it on the face or between the folds of the skin.

How to Foil Flare-Ups

Whatever treatment your doctor prescribes, you can continue the "plaque attack" on your own. Follow these hints for calmer skin.

Be a water baby. A daily 15-minute bath or shower can help reduce itching and soften scales, says Dr. Lowe. Adding a coal-tar bath solution, like Balnetar, available in drugstores, to your bathwater can provide even more itch relief.

But don't scrub-a-dub-dub. Don't scrub your skin or your scalp, says Dr. Menter. And if you're picking away scales, you may be doing more harm than good; it won't, as some people assume, help the ointments penetrate better. "Any irritation can aggravate psoriasis and make it return more quickly," says Dr. Menter.

Pat yourself dry, then lube up. Apply emollient while your skin is still damp. It's vital that you moisturize within three minutes of stepping out of the tub or shower to lock in the moisture your skin's soaked in. But avoid moisturizers formulated with fragrances or coloring agents and moisturizing gels that contain alcohol. Both can strip your skin of the water it's just absorbed.

Do the big greasy. Keeping your skin consistently moisturized with a heavy, greasy cream or ointment, like petroleum jelly or mineral oil, or a thick, heavy emollient, like Eucerin and Aquaphor, can ease scaling and inflammation and help keep psoriasis from getting worse.

Don loose, comfy duds. "Friction or pressure from clothing tends to aggravate psoriasis," says Dr. Menter. So toss out bras with straps that bind and panties with elastic waistbands that chafe, and step out of ill-fitting shoes, which can irritate the skin on your feet. Also, avoid knee-high stockings, whose elastic bands can aggravate plaques on your knees or trigger a flare-up if they rub against still-clear skin.

Stay in top form. "The better physical shape you're in, the less your psoriasis tends to flare," says Dr. Menter. Eat a healthy diet—lean meats, fish, grains and pastas, lots of fresh fruit and vegetables, low-fat yogurts and cheeses. Otherwise, disregard special restrictive diets that supposedly help clear psoriasis. "None of them have been proven to work," says Dr. Menter.

Indulge in some exercise, too. In addition to keeping you in shape, a good workout may help reduce any stress triggered by the psoriasis itself. Just make sure you wear loose-fitting workout gear without elastic waistbands that can irritate your skin.

Catch some rays—maybe. If your psoriasis responds to phototherapy, ask your doctor whether taking in some sun can further improve your skin. Don't sunbathe without clearing it with your doctor first.

If your doctor agrees, cover every exposed inch of your skin with a sunscreen that has a sun protection factor of at least 15. Sunburn can prompt severe recurrences that are more difficult to clear up.

But stay out of the sun altogether if you're fair-skinned, says Dr. Lowe. Fair-skinned people are at higher-than-average risk for skin cancer to begin with, and undergoing phototherapy increases the risk.

Don't depend on hydrocortisone. You may be wondering if over-the-counter hydrocortisone creams—made to reduce itching and inflammation—soothe psoriasis. It seems logical, but Dr. Menter claims they don't help much. "The 1 percent concentration isn't very effective for thick plaques, although it may help a bit in thin-skin areas like the groin or armpits," he says. "They're helpful in only minimal cases of psoriasis."

Ease up on alcohol. A study at the University of Michigan Medical School in Ann Arbor discovered a link between psoriasis and heavy consumption of alcohol. Heavy drinkers are three times more likely to not see results from treatment. What's more, alcohol may also trigger flare-ups. "Patients who consume too much alcohol often have more severe psoriasis," says Dr. Lowe. So if you drink,

drink in moderation—say, two glasses of wine with dinner on the weekends.

Consider some support. You might ask your doctor to refer you to the nearest support group for people with psoriasis. Dr. Lowe says, "It helps to realize that you're not alone—that there are lots of other people whose experience you can benefit from." Dr. Menter concurs. "We've seen that in group therapy situations, where patients with psoriasis can talk out their problems and thus reduce their stress level, the condition tends to improve," he says.

Protect—don't neglect. No matter how busy you get, make time to care for your skin. Pay special attention to your hands and nails. Keep your nails short, and avoid bumping or otherwise traumatizing them. Likewise, keep your hands out of dishwater and avoid exposing them to irritants like strong detergents, advises Ralph C. Daniel, M.D., clinical professor of dermatology at the University of Mississippi Medical Center in Jackson.

A Hot New Treatment for Itch Relief

One over-the-counter treatment comes from an unlikely source: Capsaicin, the ingredient that puts the bite in hot peppers, has been found to relieve the incessant itching of psoriasis. Apparently, capsaicin depletes a chemical in the body—called substance P—that transmits the itch signal to your brain, thereby lessening your urge to scratch. And less clawing may mean quicker healing.

In one study, 98 people rubbed a capsaicin cream on their flare-ups four times a day, while 99 used an inactive cream. After six weeks, 66 percent of the people who used the hot-pepper cream said their itching was gone or much improved, while only 49 percent of the other group said their itch had cooled. "Capsaicin is another approach for helping psoriasis patients, especially those who are complaining of itching," says Charles N. Ellis, M.D., professor and associate chair of the Department of Dermatology at the University of Michigan Medical School.

Capsaicin creams, available in drugstores, may burn at first, but that sensation will eventually fade. To be on the safe side, though, don't use the cream without a doctor's supervision.

CHAPTER FOURTEEN

Puffy Eyes and Dark Circles

Wake Up Those Tired Eyes

*Y*ou look tired." It's an innocent comment, even an expression of concern. But it makes you want to scream. You're dutifully in bed by 10:00 every night, but you look like you haven't slept in a week.

That's the most frustrating aspect of puffy lids, under-eye bags and dark circles—the amount of shut-eye you're getting is rarely a factor. Worse, swollen eyes and dark circles can make you look ten years older. While older women may see both conditions worsen with age, puffiness and circles are often hereditary. So younger women aren't immune.

Fortunately, you don't have to look like you're in perpetual need of a nap. You can temporarily deflate puffy eyes and hide dark circles and possibly eliminate them for good.

Puffy Eyes: Old Age—Or Just Allergies?

Minor puffiness—the kind that goes away on its own by mid-morning—is usually caused by body fluids pooling in the eye area while you're asleep, says Julius Shulman, M.D., assistant clinical professor of ophthalmology at Mount Sinai Hospital in New York City.

"But once you're up and around, these fluids will drain from your face," says Dr. Shulman.

Puffiness can also be triggered by an allergic reaction to food, dust or pollen or an allergic skin rash elsewhere on your face. If the allergy isn't treated, this temporary puffiness could become permanent, says Dr. Shulman. "Every time your lids swell from an allergic reaction, it damages the connective tissue fibers in your lids," he explains. "The more episodes of allergy and swelling you have, the looser and more puffy your lids get." So if you suspect allergies, the sooner you take steps to control the problem, the better.

Another possible culprit is eyelid dermatitis, a skin rash that riles just your lids and often affects people with sensitive skin. "Eyelid dermatitis is often caused by an allergy or sensitivity to a cosmetic or skin-care product," says Dr. Shulman, "and if the allergies keep occurring, it can result in eye bags. So stop using any product at the first sign of eye irritation." Puffy eyes may also result if you touch your eyelids after handling substances to which you're allergic, like formaldehyde in paper. So look for other possible culprits.

To treat eyelid dermatitis, your doctor may prescribe an anti-inflammatory hydrocortisone cream formulated especially for the eye area. But don't use an over-the-counter brand without consulting your doctor first: It may further irritate your eyes. More seriously, using a hydrocortisone product around your eyes for too long can cause serious eye problems, like glaucoma or cataracts. "Don't make a habit of treating even a mild case of eyelid dermatitis with hydrocortisone while you continue to use an eye pencil or moisturizer that irritates your eyes," says Dr. Shulman.

Blepharitis, an inflammation of the oil glands and lash follicles along the eyelids, is yet another cause of puffiness. Worse, this infection can cause lash loss. Not removing your eye makeup or removing it carelessly can clog the oil glands around your lids and trigger the condition. To clear the infection, your doctor may tell you to apply hot compresses or use an over-the-counter eyelid cleanser. In severe cases, she may prescribe an antibiotic ointment.

How to Send Your Bags Packing

The good news is, puffy eyes may have nothing to do with the number of birthdays you've celebrated (or bemoaned). By eliminating the cause, you can shrink excess puffiness and look years younger.

Keep your chin up—in bed. To keep fluid from pooling around your eyes, elevate your head with two or even three extra pillows, says Dr. Shulman.

Sleep on your back. Snoozing on your stomach can make body fluid head straight for your eyes, so try to learn how to sleep face-up.

Shake your salt habit. Eating too much salt can cause your body to retain water, which shows up around the thin skin around your eyes. So consider battling puffiness by switching to a low-salt diet, which is "a healthy idea in general," says Dr. Shulman.

Do Eye Gels Really Work?

If you're plagued by puffy eyes, you've probably wondered if a certain over-the-counter eye fix—the eye gel—is worth trying. The answer is maybe. While the experts are skeptical, some women say eye gels do help reduce puffiness temporarily. Many of these products contain plant extracts like witch hazel or chamomile, an herb long used to reduce puffiness.

Eye gels may offer other benefits, too. "Eye gels are wonderful under makeup," says Laura Geller, makeup artist and owner of Laura Geller Make-Up Studios, a cosmetics store in New York City. "Makeup glides on better, won't settle into PThat's because most eye gels are water-based. They contain humectants like glycerin to keep skin moist, which makes lines less noticeable, but are less greasy than oil-based eye creams.

Eye gels may also soothe tired eyes. "If your eyes get fatigued at work, patting on an eye gel over your makeup can refresh them," says Susan Nettesheim, manager of product development for face care at Pond's in Trumbull, Connecticut.

Almost every cosmetics company offers an eye gel. Two of many are Pond's Revitalizing Eye Gel and Lancome's Vivifiance Hydrating Gel. The down side: Eye gels can be expensive. Cosmetics stores have introduced their own private-label brands, however, which are often less costly.

Give your puffs the freeze. Dip a cotton ball or pad in a cup of ice water, wring it out and apply it to your lids for five to ten minutes. Or buy a gel-filled mask (sold in drugstores), freeze it, and place it on your lids for ten minutes before you start your morning routine.

Lighten up your skin-care routine. The very same oil-rich moisturizer or eye cream you're using to fight dryness could be the cause of a puffy allergic reaction. Or oily creams or cleansers could be clogging the oil glands along the edge of your eyelids, resulting in blepharitis or sties.

Try switching to water-based or oil-free skin-care products, including an oil-free eye-makeup remover, says Dr. Shulman. But stick to an oily remover if you have sensitive skin: Oil-free eye-makeup removers can irritate your eyes, triggering eyelid dermatitis.

Don't bed down in eye makeup. "It's important to remove your eye makeup thoroughly," says Dr. Shulman, especially before bed. But doing a thorough job can be trickier than you think. "Some women I see have makeup residue at the base of their lashes, even if they haven't worn makeup in a couple of days," says Dr. Shulman.

So come clean before bed, even if you're tired. "Use your remover until the tissue or cotton ball shows no trace of makeup," says Dr. Shulman. Besides keeping the oil glands in your eyelids gunk-free, you'll protect your eyes from potentially irritating flecks of mascara or shadow that may find their way into your eyes while you sleep.

Playing Down Puffiness with Makeup

Surprise: Piling on extra foundation or concealer will make bags more noticeable rather than less. Says Laura Geller, makeup artist and owner of Laura Geller Make-Up Studios, a cosmetics store in New York City, "The less makeup you use on puffy eyes, the less attention you'll call to them."

Here's how to minimize puffy eyes. First, pat on a light eye cream if you need one and if the puffiness isn't allergy related. Or you might opt for a gel formulated especially for puffy eyes. When the eye cream or gel is dry, apply your foundation, including over the puffy areas.

Finally, dust the puffy area with translucent powder to give it a matte (nonshiny) finish. Contrary to what you might have heard, a dewy finish can actually call attention to puffy areas.

If you also need to camouflage dark circles, apply concealer only to the inner corner of the under-eye area—that's where dark circles usually show up. Puffiness affects the outermost area.

When Puffs Turn to Pouches: The Fat-Zapping Option

If your eyes are constantly puffy or have formed permanent bags or pouches that defy home treatment, it may be because the normal fat around the eyes has bulged out. The condition may be inherited and show up in your teens. It could be a sign of increasing age. Then again, it could be the cumulative result of repeated allergic reactions.

Until recently, the usual solution for people who have permanently puffy eyes and are determined to get rid of them at any cost has been the traditional eye-lift, or blepharoplasty. But there is an alternative: a nonsurgical procedure called fat-melting blepharoplasty, developed by Michael Evan Sachs, M.D., director of research in the Division of Facial Plastic and Reconstructive Surgery at the New York Eye and Ear Infirmary/New York Medical College in New York City. Fat melting removes these fatty deposits by zapping them with an electrically heated needle, which evaporates the fat in seconds. Unlike traditional blepharoplasty, no cutting is necessary, and you'll usually heal within two or three days rather than the seven- to ten-day recovery period blepharoplasty requires.

But not every surgeon uses this technique. And if your fatty bags are paired with drooping skin or weakened muscle, a traditional eye-lift may be a better option for restoring a youthful appearance.

A Surgical Solution for Sleepy-Looking Lids

Drooping upper lids (which, like bags, can be inherited and appear in your twenties) can also give your eyes a puffy appearance. To perk up sagging lids, Elliott Jacobs, M.D., attending surgeon at New York Eye and Ear Infirmary and Cabrini Medical Center in New York City recommends the forehead-lift, a surgical procedure he calls a face-lift for the upper third of the face.

"The forehead-lift raises your eyebrows, which removes a lot of the extra skin and weight on the upper lids," says Dr. Jacobs. "The procedure opens the eyes dramatically without touching the upper lids at all." Best of all, there's no visible scarring—the incision is made either within your scalp or at your hairline.

Dark Circles: Lighten Them Up!

Fatigue, illness, thin skin, genetics . . . dark circles can be caused by any one of these conditions, and it may take an expert to find out which. "You can get dark circles as early as your twenties; at that age, it's usually hereditary," says Dr. Jacobs. Dark circles are also caused by hyperpigmentation (higher-than-average amounts of melanin, the substance that gives your skin its pigment), and they're especially common in people of Mediterranean descent.

Doctor's-Office Remedies for Stubborn Circles

It's easiest to hide dark circles with a concealer. But if your dark circles are severe, you might want to "erase" them permanently with one of several dermatologist-performed treatments.

KO circles with a combo treatment. Your simplest option is a dermatologist-prescribed regimen of Retin-A (topical tretinoin—the prescription vitamin A cream used to treat both fine facial wrinkles and acne) and hydroquinone, the active ingredient in over-the-counter bleaching creams, like Porcelana. "But with this treatment, you usually see a slight rather than a marked difference," says Dr. Jacobs.

A fresh approach. Melvin L. Elson, M.D., medical director of the Dermatology Center in Nashville and co-author of *The Good Look Book*, developed the "Fresh Eyes" procedure. Using a special type of collagen and a very fine needle, he places collagen between the skin and the muscle, thereby hiding the circles.

Peel circles away. Dermatologists commonly treat circles with a medium-strength trichloroacetic acid (TCA) peel or a high-strength phenol peel. Some experts feel it's safer to opt for the TCA peel, however. Phenol can cause a drastic difference in color between treated and untreated areas. This chemical can also be toxic to the heart, liver and kidneys. To be on the safe side, opt for the TCA peel—and if your circles are very dark, you might even undergo it twice.

Banish circles with surgery. Under certain lighting conditions, what may look like dark circles are actually bags, which create shadows beneath the eyes. "Remove the bag with a traditional eye-lift and the shadow goes with it," says Dr. Jacobs.

See also the chapters on eczema (chapter 10), concealers (chapter 23), allergic skin (chapter 43), chemical peels (chapter 45) and collagen injections and other filler techniques (chapter 46).

CHAPTER FIFTEEN

Sensitive Skin

Loving Care for Fussy Skin

*Y*ou won't find sensitive skin in a medical textbook. But if you have it, you know it! Sensitive skin can sting, itch and burn for seemingly no reason or break out in an irksome and all-too-noticeable rash. It can be provoked by environmental conditions like heat or cold or riled by ingredients in makeup and skin-care products. And it can be irritated by or allergic to whatever's causing these visible or invisible reactions.

As you can see, sensitive skin can be hard to pin down. But there's lots you can do to help keep temperamental skin calm and clear.

What's the Story, Anyway?

For years, most dermatologists didn't take sensitive skin too seriously. But that's changing. "Sensitive skin is common and is finally receiving serious attention," says Albert M. Kligman, M.D., Ph.D.

There's no hard-and-fast definition of sensitive skin, says Dr. Kligman. That's why you're the best judge of whether you have it. "'Anytime I put something on my skin, I break out!' is an often-heard complaint of people with sensitive skin," says Howard Murad, M.D., assistant clinical professor of dermatology at the University of

California at Los Angeles and president and CEO of Murad Skin Research Laboratories.

But according to Anthony F. Fransway, M.D., assistant professor of dermatology at the University of South Florida in Tampa, sensitive skin has certain characteristics: It's easily irritated by environmental factors like dust and pet dander, is fertile ground for other conditions like acne and eczema and reacts to certain cosmetic ingredients with irritation or allergy. Sensitive skin is likely to be even more sensitive if it's affected by another skin condition like seborrheic dermatitis or rosacea (pronounced ro-ZAY-shuh), adds Dr. Murad.

Rashes, Breakouts and Bumps: Now You See 'Em, Now You Don't

Sensitive skin most often stings and burns from reactions you can feel but not see—a condition dermatologists call subjective irritation. "With subjective irritation, the skin looks normal," says Dr. Kligman. Sensitive skin can also break out or turn red, dry and chapped from heat, cold or various environmental factors that other folks tolerate well.

Sensitive skin can also erupt in hives or contact dermatitis—red, itchy rashes often triggered by ingredients in skin-care products, usually fragrances and preservatives. Irritant contact dermatitis commonly stings and appears scaly, dry or chapped, while allergic contact dermatitis is generally bumpy and itchy.

Most cosmetic-induced skin reactions are irritations, not allergies. While a patch test can determine whether an allergy to a cosmetic ingredient is triggering your rashes or breakouts, no one has come up with a similar test for irritants. So you'll have to find out what's riling your skin by determining what isn't—in other words, a product-by-product process of elimination.

One woman was completely perplexed as to why the skin under her eyes (a particularly vulnerable area for many people with sensitive skin) was dry, flaky and cracked. She finally figured out that silver from the label of her "sensitive skin formula moisturizer" was being transferred from the bottle to her eyes via her fingers every time she applied the moisturizer to her face. Once she made the connection, the solution was simple: She applied a strip of clear plastic packing tape over the label, and the problem disappeared almost immediately.

Stressed-Out Skin? Take a Look around You

Winter cold, summer heat, dry air and dust can all provoke sensitive skin. So try to calm your hide by adjusting your environment.

Come in from the cold. "Your skin feels more sensitive during the winter because it gets dry and dehydrated," says Dr. Murad. If cold weather aggravates your skin, follow the routine for dry skin on page 191. You might also use a humidifier to help keep the air—and your skin—moist.

Beat the heat. Your own perspiration can irritate your skin, so try to keep your environment cool, says Dr. Fransway. But don't park yourself too close to a fan or air conditioner. "High-airflow environments can have a terribly drying effect on skin," he says.

Also, consider skipping foundation in hot weather, says Dr. Fransway. Face makeup can block your pores, prevent your perspiration from evaporating and possibly trigger a breakout.

Keep your guard up. House dust, molds, grasses, mildew and pet dander (particles on fur) can make sensitive skin go haywire. So keep an eye out for potential trigger factors.

Soften your water. Use a water softener if you live in a hard-water area, suggests Dr. Fransway. Removing excess minerals from the water may improve its rinsability, washing away cleanser residue that—if left on your face—can rile sensitive skin.

Softer water can also help in the laundry room. "Using towels that

Shun These Sensitizers

Virtually any ingredient in a skin-care product has the potential to aggravate sensitive skin. But be especially wary of these common irritants.

→ Quaternium-15 (a preservative)
→ Benzoic acid (a preservative)
→ Parabens (a preservative)
→ Sorbic acid (a preservative)
→ Benzyl alcohol (a solvent in perfumes)
→ Lactic acid (an alpha hydroxy acid)

contain detergent residue can irritate your skin," says Amy New-burger, M.D., associate clinical professor of dermatology at the College of Physicians and Surgeons of Columbia University and assistant attending physician at Presbyterian Hospital in New York City.

Skin-Friendly Bath and Shower Strategies

Bath products and even water itself can irritate sensitive skin—but not if you come clean right. So try these tips the next time you step into the tub or shower.

Make it quick. Keep baths and showers short (ten minutes or less) and tepid rather than long and steamy. Hot water can strip skin of its natural oils, causing dryness and irritation.

Heal with oatmeal. A colloidal oatmeal product like Aveeno (which is pulverized to extra-fine particles so it stays suspended in water) can help soothe itchiness and irritation and leaves behind an invisible, protective film on the surface of the skin. Almost as important: Colloidal oatmeal won't clog your drain.

Oiling up's up to you. Some dermatologists suggest adding mineral or cottonseed oil to your bath if you have sensitive skin. But Dr. Newburger says oils don't help. "First, they make the tub slippery. Second, they float on top of the water, so the only time the oil gets on your skin is when you get out of the tub—not enough to make it worthwhile."

Whether to use oil is up to you. But never use scented bath oil, cubes, salts or gels. Fragrances are well-known sensitizers and often cause sensitive skin to flare.

Towel off gently. When you step out of the tub and shower, pat, rather than rub, your skin dry. Then immediately slather on a thick moisturizer like Eucerin Plus, Moisturel or Dermasil to seal in the moisture your skin has absorbed.

Shave sensibly. Chemical hair removers, waxing and electrolysis are likely to irritate sensitive skin. Dr. Murad recommends shaving your legs and underarms with a shaving gel, which is less drying than a regular shaving cream. Never shave dry, bare skin—it can raise an itchy rash or a crop of bumps. "If you don't have a shaving gel, use an unscented, nonsoap bar," says Dr. Newburger.

Just-shaved skin can flare if subjected to other products. "Any ingredient you're sensitive to, you're going to be more sensitive to after shaving," says Dr. Murad. So if you use a sunless tanner on your legs, apply it the night before, not after, you shave. But shave your underarms at night so your skin can recover before you apply antiperspirant in the morning.

Stick to the Basics

The fewer skin-care products you use, the calmer your skin is likely to be. So use only products you absolutely, positively need. "Generally, you need a cleanser, a moisturizer and a sunscreen you can use without a problem," says Dr. Newburger.

Cleanser-selection tips. Harsh deodorant or antibacterial soaps can dry skin—especially sensitive skin—to the bone. Use a soap-free, superfatted, unscented bar like Dove or Cetaphil, a gentle soap substitute. Cetaphil can be used without water, which can be a boon for sensitive skin. "Even water can irritate sensitive skin, so using a tissue-off rather than a rinse-away cleanser may be easier on your skin," says Dr. Murad. You might also try RoC's Gel Cleansing Wash, part of the RoC skin-care line, available in drugstores. "It's a wonderful line for sensitive skin," says Dr. Newburger.

Avoid harsh skin-care products like abrasive facial pads or grainy face and body scrubs, which can strip away the protective top layer of skin—your defensive armor against heat, cold, pollution, irritants and other antagonists.

If you have sensitive skin, the eyes require extra vigilance to avoid nasty reactions. Says Dr. Fransway, "Your eyelids are so thin and so sensitive to irritants that they often become dry, scaly and itchy." So avoid using harsh soaps and alcohol-based astringents and toners.

Cleanse away eye makeup with an oily remover rather than an oil-free product. Whatever product you use, gently stroke away eye makeup with a cotton swab or pad. Scrubbing with a tissue or washcloth can irritate your lids.

Choosing a moisturizer. Along with hydrating your skin's top layer, a moisturizer acts as a defensive barrier between your skin and your makeup. Dr. Newburger suggests trying one of the moisturizers in the RoC skin-care line or a rose water and glycerin moisturizer, which contains just two basic ingredients. You might also use plain old petroleum jelly, says Dr. Kligman. Too greasy for daytime, you say? Not at all. Just use a very thin layer.

If you've been wanting to try a moisturizer formulated with glycolic acid, an alpha hydroxy acid (AHA), you can, say experts. In general, sensitive skin can tolerate moisturizers formulated with these fruit-derived acids that slough off dead, complexion-dulling skin cells. But before you apply an AHA-enhanced product on your face, perform a use test on your arm (see below). The chance of irri-

Is Natural Better? Maybe Not

Skin-care products made with plant extracts, fruits and vegetables and other natural ingredients often look and smell great. But if you have sensitive skin, they might not feel so great. According to Anthony F. Fransway, M.D., assistant professor of dermatology at the University of South Florida in Tampa, some natural ingredients may irritate sensitive skin or even trigger allergic reactions. "There's no question in my mind that many ingredients in so-called natural skin-care products have a certain sensitizing potential that synthetic products may not," says Dr. Fransway.

If you have sensitive skin, Dr. Fransway recommends avoiding all natural products, especially those formulated with royal jelly or propolis (obtained from honey bees and often found in "rejuvenating" skin treatments or wrinkle creams), melaleuca (obtained from a tree native to Australia and sometimes found in products that heal cuts and burns) and—surprisingly—aloe vera, the gel of the aloe vera plant known for its skin-healing qualities. "Aloe vera can be terribly irritating to sensitive skin," says Dr. Fransway. He also suggests avoiding aromatherapy, which uses plant and flower oils in massage and other skin treatments. "Fragrances cause between 5 and 10 percent of all contact allergies," says Dr. Fransway.

Man-made ingredients can rile sensitive skin, too, says Dr. Fransway, and many people who use natural products are quite happy with them. "But just because a product is natural doesn't necessarily mean it's safe or good for you," he says. "Besides, there isn't a lot of proof that these products work."

tation depends on the product's pH, AHA concentration and other ingredients, says Dr. Murad. You might also avoid products containing lactic acid, an AHA that's been known to irritate sensitive skin.

Sun-protection selection. Choose products formulated with physical-barrier sunscreens like zinc oxide or titanium dioxide. If you still think of zinc oxide as clown makeup, think again. Zinc oxide isn't the unattractive white paste it used to be. Like titanium dioxide, zinc oxide can now be micronized (reduced to virtually invisible particles). Some companies add zinc oxide and titanium dioxide to chemical sunscreens, however. So if you have sensitive skin, make sure the product you choose is 100 percent chemical-free, like Almay's Fragrance-Free Suncare SPF 30+ Sensitive Skin Formula or Neutrogena's Chemical-Free Sunblocker SPF 17.

Avoid products formulated with chemical sunscreens like PABA (para-aminobenzoic acid) or the cinnamate or oxybenzone families of sunscreens, all of which can irritate sensitive skin.

Strip Down Your Makeup

You don't necessarily have to give up wearing makeup just because you have sensitive skin. You just have to find the right products. These tips can help.

Head for the hypoallergenic. Many cosmetics companies, including Almay, Physicians Formula, Clinique and Elizabeth Arden, make hypoallergenic makeup, which contains fewer skin-irritating preservatives and fragrances. But even hypoallergenic products aren't completely safe. They're just less likely to rile sensitive skin. Says Dr. Newburger, "Hypoallergenic is not necessarily hypo-irritating."

Use an oil-based foundation. In Dr. Newburger's experience, oil-based foundations are less likely to provoke sensitive skin than water-based products because they contain fewer and different preservatives.

Oil-rich foundations are fine for both dry and oily skin, says Dr. Newburger. She suggests Countess Isserlyn by Alexandra de Markoff. And if you're prone to breakouts, choose a water-based over an oil-free foundation: "Your skin's natural oils will make an oil-free foundation darken on your skin after a few hours," says Dr. Newburger.

Put your makeup to the test. You can determine whether a new foundation or blusher will rile your skin before you use it, says Dr. Fransway. Here's how: Dab a small amount of the product on your inner forearm twice a day for a week to see if your skin reacts.

This test, called the use test, isn't foolproof, however. Some ingredients irritate the skin on your face, while others affect only the thin, delicate skin of your eyelids. Test only moisturizers and face cosmetics, says Dr. Fransway. Avoid testing eye shadow, mascara, eyeliner or hair-care products, which are more likely to irritate sensitive skin.

Don't stray from tried-and-true products. Once you find makeup your skin can handle, stick with it. "Some women find cosmetics that agree with their skin but then want to try new ones," says Alexander Fisher, M.D., clinical professor of dermatology at New York University Medical Center in New York City. But when the urge to experiment strikes, it's safer to try a new hairstyle than a new foundation.

If all else fails... If you've tried all the suggestions in this chapter and they've failed to calm your skin or if you suspect a cosmetic or skin-care product of causing your rashes or breakouts, consult a dermatologist. She may ask that you bring in all your skin-care products to try to sleuth out a possible culprit. "One ingredient may be causing the trouble," says Dr. Fransway.

Cosmetic Procedures Aren't Off-Limits

It's worth emphasizing that women with sensitive skin must be doubly vigilant when considering cosmetic procedures. But according to Dr. Kligman, many cosmetic treatments are open to people with sensitive skin. "A dermatologist can prescribe Retin-A (topical tretinoin—the vitamin A–derived treatment for wrinkles) in a lower concentration," says Dr. Kligman. Sensitive-skinned people can also peel away fine lines and sun damage with a glycolic acid or trichloroacetic acid (TCA) facial peel, says Dr. Kligman.

An important caveat: Tell your dermatologist you have sensitive skin before you undergo any cosmetic procedure, advises Dr. Klingman. "If you tell a dermatologist, 'I think I have sensitive skin,' she might give you a 20 percent glycolic acid peel rather than 70 percent," he says.

See also the chapters on dandruff and related problems (chapter 9), eczema (chapter 10) and dry skin (chapter 34).

CHAPTER SIXTEEN

Stretch Marks

Smoothing Skin under Pressure

As far as beauty pet peeves are concerned, stretch marks rank right up there with blemishes and cellulite. Especially exasperating is the fact that stretch marks can show up on your hips, thighs, breasts or buttocks even if you diligently work out, eat right and take other steps to help ensure clear, smooth skin elsewhere on your body.

The good news is, stretch marks don't necessarily have to leave their mark on your skin. You may be able to control them if you catch them early enough in the game. And if you can't eliminate stretch marks, you can do the next best thing: conceal them.

Anatomy of a Stretch Mark

Stretch marks result when collagen, a protein substance that gives your skin its elasticity, tears away from the skin's connective fibers; the marks most often appear when the deeper layers of the skin, the dermis, expand, as after a large weight gain (and subsequent loss), or during pregnancy. In fact, about one out of three women who have given birth get stretch marks, says Albert M. Kligman, M.D., Ph.D.

But take comfort. If you developed stretch marks during pregnancy, there's a good possibility heredity's to blame. "To some degree, you can avoid stretch marks by watching your weight. But whether you'll get stretch marks when you get pregnant depends on your genetic makeup," says Stephen M. Purcell, D.O., chairman of the Division of Dermatology at the Philadelphia College of Osteopathic Medicine.

Stretch marks can also be caused by a growth spurt in adolescence or the use of hydrocortisone creams, which are often prescribed for serious skin problems and which can thin the skin. So don't use a potent steroid cream on a minor irritation.

Stretch marks don't start out as wavy white bands on unsuspecting skin, however. They debut as tender and somewhat painful purplered lines. This inflammatory stage can last four or five months. The purplish marks eventually fade, leaving behind thin, almost invisible

The Cocoa Butter Challenge

Does rubbing cocoa butter on stretch marks really help eliminate them? No, says Albert M. Kligman, M.D., Ph.D., who has assembled an entire list of potions and treatments that supposedly fade stretch marks. "The Chinese use herbs. The Japanese use different oils. Some American salons use electrical treatments that shock the tissue. But most of these treatments have no scientific basis at all and just don't work."

So whether you're using cocoa butter, olive oil or even vitamin E—a popular folk cure for stretch marks—"don't expect these ingredients to fade stretch marks at any stage," says Dr. Kligman.

What may help is massage. Stephen M. Purcell, D.O., chairman of the Division of Dermatology at the Philadelphia College of Osteopathic Medicine, says that there's been some anecdotal evidence that massaging stretch marks with these types of oils or creams has somewhat improved their appearance. *Anecdotal evidence* means that people who've tried it swear it works, but researchers have not been able to prove it in laboratory studies. "But what's probably working is the massage," says Dr. Purcell.

silvery gray stretch marks or wider, deeper, whiter marks. "Once stretch marks reach this stage, they're technically scars," says Dr. Kligman.

No reason to fret. Body concealers like Dermablend and Covermark can hide stretch marks quite effectively, especially if they haven't left indentations in your skin.

Retin-A to the Rescue—Again

If you catch stretch marks in the earliest, formative stage, you may be able to squelch them altogether. Retin-A (topical tretinoin), the synthetic form of vitamin A used to treat facial lines and acne, can prevent stretch marks still in the inflammatory stage from developing into scars.

Retin-A works by stimulating your skin's production of collagen and interrupting the inflammatory process that breaks down the deeper layers of skin, or dermis, explains Dr. Kligman. But you need to act fast: Once stretch marks become scars, nothing—including Retin-A—will budge them.

Dermatologists treat stretch marks that are just developing with a high-strength concentration of Retin-A, even more potent than what's used on facial lines. While some doctors prescribe a nightly application, Dr. Kligman says it's better to rub your marks with Retin-A twice a day if you can tolerate the irritation. Treatment lasts about three to six months. Dr. Purcell's patients supplement their Retin-A treatment by moisturizing their marks each morning with glycolic or lactic acid, two members of the alpha hydroxy acid (AHA) group. AHAs, also used in light facial peels, appear to slough off the outer layer of skin cells and increase cell turnover, leaving smoother, fresher skin behind.

Though you may eventually love the results, don't expect to enjoy the treatment itself, warns Dr. Kligman. "You're not going to like it," he says. "You're going to say it stings and burns and peels." Still, notes Dr. Purcell, "Studies have shown that patients who didn't get that irritated response didn't do as well." In other words, no pain, no gain.

If you're pregnant, don't begin Retin-A therapy until after you give birth. Experts are still divided as to whether this drug could cause birth defects. The experts' advice: Talk it over with your obstetrician.

See also the chapter on concealers (chapter 23).

CHAPTER SEVENTEEN

Sunburn

Instant Relief for Pain and Peeling

*U*h-oh. Despite your best intentions, you have sunburn. Perhaps you forgot to reapply sunscreen after a swim. Or you fell asleep in the sun. Or you exposed your winter-pale skin to the sun for only an hour to perk up your complexion. Now you have a sun-induced glow that's a little bit more colorful—and painful—than you expected.

The Sunburn Blues: Too Little, Too Late

Sunburn is a delayed reaction to sun exposure and an actual wound to your skin. A sunburn's pain and inflammation begin 3 to 5 hours after the damage has been done and peak after about 15 hours. That's why it's so easy to be taken by surprise—you may not feel like you're burning until much later.

Ironically, sunburn is your body's attempt to protect your skin and minimize further damage. How severely you burn depends on how long you spend in the sun and your skin type. The fairer your skin, the worse you will burn. But even darker skin can turn stop-sign red. Making matters worse, sunburn breaks down your skin's store of elastin and collagen, the materials that give skin its firmness and elasticity, causing wrinkles.

But sunburn isn't just unattractive—it's dangerous. The more sunburns you get, the greater your risk for developing skin cancer. A Scottish study found that people who had at least three severe sunburns in their lives increased their risk of skin cancer. But according to Karen E. Burke, M.D., Ph.D., attending physician at Cabrini Medical Center in New York City and adjunct clinical member of Scripps Clinic and Research Foundation in California, just one burn can up your chances of skin cancer, even if it's been years since you fried yourself to a crisp. "A single, blistering sunburn as a child doubles the risk of skin cancer in adulthood," says Dr. Burke.

Sunburns can also weaken your body's ability to battle disease. Research by Kevin D. Cooper, M.D., associate professor and director of the Immunodermatology Unit at the University of Michigan at Ann Arbor, has shown that even mild sunburns can reduce your immune system's ability to react in self-defense.

Fast Fixes for the French-Fried

Since most of your sunburn's pain, redness and inflammation will probably disappear in a day or two, treatments for mild sunburn involve getting you through the immediate agony. The following steps will ease your burn and jump-start your skin's healing process.

Keep cool. Drape yourself in cool, moist towels, suggests Rodney S. W. Basler, M.D., head of a task force on sports medicine and assistant professor of dermatology at the University of Nebraska Medical Center in Omaha. He suggests applying, then removing, the towels every half-hour for four or five hours or until bedtime, when you should apply a soothing cream or ointment (see below). You might also soak in a tub of cool water to which you've added baking soda or a colloidal oatmeal bath product like Aveeno. Let yourself air-dry!

Make like a camel. Sunburn really dehydrates your body, so replenish lost fluids by drinking plenty of water. Upping your fluid intake may also indirectly soothe sunburn pain. After inflammation, dehydration causes the most discomfort, says Dr. Basler.

Kiss pain good-bye with aloe. Soothing sizzled skin with the gel of the aloe vera plant is an effective sunburn remedy. Aloe contains lectin, an aspirin-like compound that seems to relieve the sting of a sunburn, says John P. Heggers, M.D., professor of surgery in the Division of Plastic and Reconstructive Surgery, professor of microbiology at the University of Texas Medical Branch and director of clin-

Don't Get Fooled Again

Photosensitivity occurs when certain drugs, cosmetic fragrances or foods make your skin more likely to burn when it's exposed to sunlight.

There are two kinds of photosensitivity reactions: photoallergy and phototoxicity. A photoallergy, which triggers your immune system to rile your skin, is characterized by an itchy rash. Ironically, PABA (para-aminobenzoic acid), a chemical sunscreen, is a known skin allergen. Phototoxicity doesn't make your immune system turn traitor, but it does cause a burning sensation and a rash that, within hours, resembles a bad sunburn. The rash peels within a few days.

Either way, a surprise sunburn warrants further investigation. Scrutinize this checklist of common ingredients. Then consult your doctor for help in testing the likely offender (or offenders), so you can steer clear of the culprits in the future.

- → Psoralens (a substance found in celery, carrots and the oil on the peel of limes)
- → Fragrances in cosmetics, including musk ambrette, balsam of Peru and oil of bergamot
- → PABA
- → Antibiotics like tetracycline and doxycycline
- → Thiazides (diuretics often prescribed for high blood pressure)
- → Some antifungals, including griseofulvin
- → Phenothiazines (psychiatric drugs)

ical microbiology at the Shriners Burns Institute in Galveston.

While you can use the gel from a live aloe plant by snipping off a spike, Dr. Heggers's research has shown that using a concentrated extract found in the cream-based product Dermaide, available in drugstores, is almost twice as effective as gel used straight from the plant.

Be kind to a burned kisser. If your lips burned—and they probably did, as they contain little pigment to protect them—smooth them with petroleum jelly alone or over a dab or so of a hydrocortisone cream, suggests Dr. Basler. Don't use a fruit-flavored or other cosmetic lip balm. "They may contain perfume or other alcohol-based ingredients that could further irritate your lips," adds Dr. Heggers.

Don't wear makeup. While you can use moisturizer, says Dr. Basler, don't wear makeup to hide your sunburned skin. "If at all possible, you should avoid wearing makeup for two days after a burn," says Dr. Basler. If you happen to be a Broadway actress or are simply going out for a special night on the town, wear makeup sparingly. Adds Dr. Basler, "Before you put on your makeup, apply a very thin layer of 1 percent hydrocortisone cream—it will act as a barrier."

Stop the hurt with hydrocortisone. An over-the-counter cream containing 1 percent hydrocortisone, an anti-inflammatory ingredient, will ease your burn's swelling and pain. Dr. Basler suggests you top the hydrocortisone with a rich emollient, like Aquaphor, Eucerin or petroleum jelly, to enhance the hydrocortisone's effect and to hydrate burned skin even more.

Don't numb out. While some doctors recommend over-the-counter local anesthetics like Solarcaine to relieve the pain of a sunburn, others advise against using them. "Local anesthetics should not be used," says Albert M. Kligman, M.D., Ph.D. Benzocaine, the common ingredient in these products, can sensitize your skin, triggering an allergic reaction potentially worse than the sunburn itself.

Reach for the aspirin. If you take aspirin immediately, this anti-inflammatory may cut a burn's redness and swelling and will definitely help soothe the pain.

If you're allergic to aspirin, doctors recommend trying acetaminophen instead; it doesn't have the anti-inflammatory action aspirin does, but it will relieve some discomfort.

Scorched Skin Is Serious Business

If your sunburned skin is extremely tender, painful, swollen or blistered or if you develop fever, chills, dizziness or nausea within 12 hours of sun exposure, see your doctor or go to the nearest emergency room. You may need antibiotics for severe blistering or corticosteroids for the dizziness and nausea.

You should also head to a doctor if your skin sloughs off or appears infected, if your burn was caused by photosensitivity (see "Don't Get Fooled Again" on page 91) or if it turns a deep purple red by the second day—all signs of deep skin damage.

CHAPTER EIGHTEEN

Varicose Veins

Beautiful Legs Can Be Yours Again

Thinking of trading in your tennis whites for black tights, or your golf shorts for hip waders? If bluish veins have started popping out behind your knees—or if tiny red spider veins are sprouting on your thighs—you have a classic (though probably mild) case of varicose veins.

No need to feel vain if the appearance of these unsightly vessels disturbs you, especially if they're accompanied by the tired, achy leg fatigue that can keep you away from the activities and clothes you love. Here's how to get a leg up on varicose veins.

Legs under Pressure

Unfair, but true: Women are plagued with varicose veins four times as often as men. These vessels appear when the veins in your legs can't pump blood back up to your heart: Either the vein walls weaken or your veins' flaplike valves—which are supposed to shut if your blood starts to flow back into your legs—fail. Either way, your blood pools in your leg veins, which causes them to bulge. And they hurt.

Varicose veins are often inherited, but they're also brought on by anything that increases the pressure on your leg veins: standing up or sitting down for long periods (which causes blood to settle in your

Work Out to Your Heart's (and Legs') Content

Don't let varicose veins stand in the way of your daily workout. Just choose an activity that doesn't encourage the unsightly vessels. "Don't overlook walking, which pumps up your muscles, squeezes your veins and pushes blood back up to your heart," says Walter P. de Groot, M.D., a vascular surgeon at the Swedish Medical Center in Seattle and past president of the North American Society of Phlebology.

Activities to pursue:
→ Swimming
→ Walking
→ Bicycling
→ Leg lifts

Activities to avoid:
→ High-impact exercise (aerobics, especially step aerobics)
→ Running (especially on inclines)
→ Stair-climbing
→ Jumping jacks

legs), carrying too much weight, certain types of exercise, pregnancy (the expanding uterus puts pressure on pelvic and leg veins) and hormonal changes triggered by the Pill.

Tips for Lovelier, Livelier Legs

Most efforts to manage varicose veins attempt to prevent blood from pooling in your legs and pump it back up toward your heart. Here's how you can help it on its way—and help prevent leg veins from worsening.

Give yourself some support. Wearing support hose, available at most drugstores, keeps your blood from pooling in your legs. For heavy-duty support, ask your doctor about custom-fitted, more heavily elasticized hose.

Take off the tight stuff. Don't wear tight panty hose or constricting foundation garments like panty girdles; they can cut off your circulation.

Get moving. Don't sit or stand for long periods. If you sit at a desk all day, take frequent breaks to get up and walk around.

Kick up your heels. To help your blood make the return trip to your heart, elevate your legs above the level of your heart for 10 to 15 minutes three or four times a day.

Get back into circulation. Getting regular exercise will keep your blood circulating nicely. Even a 20-minute daily walk is fine. But avoid high-impact aerobics and stair-climbing: They stress your vascular system, can lead to valve damage and may cause varicose veins in genetically predisposed people. (See "Work Out to Your Heart's (and Legs') Content" for good-for-your-legs workouts.)

Take special care if you're expecting. Varicose veins are especially likely to appear or worsen when you're pregnant, so follow the tips above. Also, don't gain too much weight, wear special maternity support hose and sleep on your side to keep your uterus from putting unnecessary pressure on underlying blood vessels.

Chill on the Pill. If you first noticed varicose or spider veins after you started taking birth control pills, take notice: The high levels of estrogen in estrogen-based oral contraceptives are associated with the development of varicose veins.

Makeup That Plays Down Leg Veins

Minor spider or varicose veins are easily camouflaged with special body concealers like Dermablend and Covermark. To use these products successfully, follow these expert tips.

Go for the package deal. Body concealers often need to be used with a powder—usually called a setting or sealing powder—that waterproofs the concealer and keeps it from rubbing off on your clothing. And since these concealers are made to last, you'll also want to use your brand's companion remover. When it comes to camouflaging skin imperfections, it doesn't pay to skimp.

Use the right tool. Apply the concealer with a small, synthetic-hair makeup brush, says Laura Geller, makeup artist and owner of Laura Geller Make-Up Studios, a cosmetics store in New York City. "This way, you only have to 'paint' the vein itself," she says. After you conceal the imperfection, blend the concealer with a sponge, "leaving the heaviest amount of concealer on the vein itself and sheering out the edges along the sides of the vein so the product gradually blends into your skin," says Geller.

Don't overconceal. You can't make large, bulging varicose veins disappear with concealer, no matter how much you use. In fact, using too much concealer may draw attention to the problem.

Sclerotherapy: No Pain, No Vein

If self-care isn't satisfactory and your veins are severely distended, your doctor will probably suggest sclerotherapy, an in-office procedure that works without pain or scarring. As medical procedures go, it's relatively safe and convenient: Sclerotherapy takes less than an hour, and in most cases, you'll be up and around immediately.

Here's how sclerotherapy works. Your doctor injects the affected vessel (or vessels) with a special solution, which irritates the vein, causing it to shrivel and close off. You might feel a bit of cramping or tenderness immediately afterward. And to make sure the vein gets as much exposure to the solution as possible, you may have to wear support hose for a couple of days to a few weeks. But the vein itself will completely disappear in two to six weeks.

For the best results, you might need to undergo sclerotherapy more than once, says Walter P. de Groot, M.D., a vascular surgeon at the Swedish Medical Center in Seattle and past president of the North American Society of Phlebology. "Some patients want perfect results—and we can come very close," he says.

Sclerotherapy's not without complications, however. You may experience browning (blood, actually), a localized skin reaction that's usually caused by using a too-strong solution, or matting—dilated capillaries at or near the injected area. Browning usually fades in a few months and rarely lasts more than a year. Experts don't always know what causes matting, but the capillaries usually disappear on their own: Give it six months, says Neil Sadick, M.D., assistant clinical professor of dermatology at Cornell University Medical College in New York City. Capillaries that linger after that can be re-treated.

Less commonly, sclerotherapy can cause ulcers at the site of the injection, and in extremely rare cases, you could be allergic to the sclerotherapy solution. Also, don't undergo sclerotherapy if you're pregnant or nursing. Experts don't yet know whether the solutions used in the procedure affect either the fetus or breast milk.

Surgery: A Sometimes Solution

If your varicose veins are very large, you may need to have them surgically removed. But surgery is usually quick. Most likely, you'll leave the hospital or outpatient treatment center the same day and recover in a few days.

In the most common type of vein surgery, ambulatory phlebectomy, the surgeon makes multiple incisions and removes the varicose vein or veins. The incisions are tiny—a few millimeters long—so scarring is virtually invisible.

Some varicose veins are caused by pressure at the junction of the two veins—the saphenous vein closest to the skin and the more important femoral vein. If this is the case, your surgeon may perform another minor surgical procedure—ligation and division—to disconnect the two veins. Some surgeons may also remove part of the saphenous vein from groin to knee, but it's rarely necessary, says Dr. de Groot. This high-speed procedure takes only 30 to 45 minutes and often reduces or even completely eliminates the varicose veins. Your doctor can treat any lingering veins with sclerotherapy a month after surgery.

There may even be a quicker treatment for varicose veins. The Food and Drug Administration is now reviewing a new laserlike technology called Photoderm, which treats leg veins that are less than the thickness of a pencil and which may reduce side effects like browning and matting.

See also the chapters on cosmetic surgery (chapter 47) and concealers (chapter 23).

CHAPTER NINETEEN

Warts

Get Them Off Your Hands for Good

There's nothing like a wart to spoil the elegant appearance of a good manicure, or to detract from the beauty of otherwise smooth, pretty hands. And if warts have made their way to your face or popped up between your toes or on the soles of your feet, they're even less welcome.

These stubborn little growths—caused by an equally stubborn, if usually harmless, virus—can be difficult to get rid of. But you can win the war of the warts. Here's how.

A Toad-ally Awful Affliction

Warts are abnormal growths caused by the human papillomavirus (HPV), a hardy family of about 60 varieties that sprouts warts almost anywhere on your body. You'll probably recognize a wart when you see one. The average wart has a rough, scaly surface with definite borders and is skin-colored or slightly darker than the surrounding skin. Yet there are noticeable variations. So-called common warts are scaly, rough and raised and usually appear on your hands and fingers. Palmar warts are scaly, thick, callus-covered warts that show up on your palms. Flat warts, usually found on your legs or face, are tiny, nearly flat and nonscaly; you may get dozens of them at a time. Plantar warts, which sprout on the soles of your feet, can be extremely painful, making walking or even standing difficult.

The wart virus is highly contagious and thrives in warm, moist places; you can pick up a virus from a towel or by walking barefoot at your health club, or by direct contact with someone who has the virus. The virus can even sneak through a cut or abrasion, like a paper cut on your finger. And since the virus can survive for quite some time, you might not spot a wart until months after you're exposed.

So why do some of us get warts while others don't? It may have to do with how often you're exposed to the virus or the fact that the skin on which the wart appears was somehow irritated. Picking a hangnail, for example, can increase your chances of getting a wart on your finger. Or you may be innately susceptible to warts, the way some people catch a cold or develop athlete's foot more easily than others.

Often, warts disappear on their own. "Half to two-thirds of all warts will go away in two years without treatment," says Karl R. Beutner, M.D., assistant clinical professor of dermatology at the University of California at San Francisco. But that means a third of all warts won't do a disappearing act, and two years might be too long to wait. And there's no way to know whether your warts will be limited to one or two, multiply to four and stop or keep multiplying indefinitely.

Don't Pick at That Wart!

If there's one thing you shouldn't do when you have a wart, it's pick at it. So avoid the temptation to snip, shave, pick at or try to remove any growth yourself, especially if you aren't sure of what it is. The more you worry warts, the more you encourage them to spread.

Nibbling at them is even worse. "People who bite their warts can get them on their lips," says Karl R. Beutner, M.D., assistant clinical professor of dermatology at the University of California at San Francisco. Besides, it's gross.

Hand-to-Hand Wart Warfare

A wart is a wily enemy; no method of removal is guaranteed because there's no way to make sure you've killed all the virus within and around the wart, along with the wart itself. "And even if you decide to do something about your warts, there are no quick cures," says Dr. Beutner. But don't get discouraged—try these on-your-own remedies.

Over-the-counter wart removers. These liquids or pads formulated with salicylic acid may work, especially on small warts, and they're inexpensive. But these products can take months to dissolve larger warts, if they work at all. "Many warts that go away with these removers probably would have gone away on their own," says Dr. Beutner.

Some of these products might even harm your skin. Says Glenn Gastwirth, D.P.M., deputy executive director of the American Podiatric Medical Association in Bethesda, Maryland, "Liquid wart removers can burn through healthy tissue and leave an open sore that can get infected—all without ever reaching the deep core of the wart."

A few cautions: Never use these products on your face or on warts with hair or moles. And if you have poor circulation or diabetes, don't self-treat your warts at all; you may not be able to feel whether the remover is eating through your skin or causing an infection.

Smother your warts. You may be able to wipe out a wart by covering it with tape for about three weeks. "You wrap it with multiple layers of duct tape or real cloth adhesive tape for 6½ days at a time, then remove it for half a day and repeat the process," says Dr. Beutner. "Patients tell me that it works."

Doctor's-Office Wart Cures

Which wart-removal method your doctor uses depends on where the warts are located, how widespread they are and the pros and cons of each treatment.

Sometimes the prime consideration is recovery time. If you have a plantar wart, you'll be able to walk sooner if you have it chemically removed rather than cut away. Scarring is yet another factor. The more aggressive the treatment—lasers, electrosurgery and curettage (see below)—the greater the risk of scarring, says Dr. Beutner.

Warts around the fingernails are especially difficult to treat, says Paul Kechijian, M.D., clinical associate professor of dermatology and chief of the nail section at the New York University Medical Center in New York City. These warts are inherently more resistant to treatment, and there's usually more than one to contend with. What's more, any of the treatments below could penetrate the nail and injure the nail root. "You don't want to cure your warts while permanently damaging your nails," says Dr. Kechijian.

If multiple warts have sprouted around your nails, "don't aggressively treat them," advises Dr. Kechijian—first try less drastic treatments, like salicylic acid or freezing, which are discussed below. They may then shrink enough to remove surgically.

But regardless of which method you choose, you may have to have the wart treated more than once to completely kill the virus.

Patch it up. A skin patch called Trans-Ver-Sal delivers a dose of salicylic acid that's absorbed by your wart. You stick on a patch at night and remove it in the morning. But according to Dr. Beutner, these patches may not work better than over-the-counter salicylic plasters or paint-on removers—and the treatment is more expensive. And don't expect overnight results; you may have to patch up your wart for six weeks.

As with over-the-counter salicylic treatments, these patches (available only by prescription) shouldn't be used by people with diabetes or poor circulation.

Freeze warts away. Your doctor may pare down the wart to expose its capillaries and swab or spray it with liquid nitrogen; the intense cold causes the wart to blister, scab and fall off. "Essentially, liquid nitrogen gives the wart frostbite and kills it," says Dr. Beutner. The freezing itself takes about 30 seconds; you might feel pain for a few minutes, then discomfort for up to three days. The down side: It's possible that you'll need to undergo the treatment more than once. The up side: Freezing is least likely to leave a scar.

Burn off the bumps. In electrosurgery, the doctor gives you a local anesthetic and then uses an electric current to destroy the wart by burning it away. "It 'cooks' the wart," says Dr. Beutner. "And it smells like burning chicken feathers." This treatment is also likely to cause scarring.

Cut warts away. In curettage, your doctor uses an instrument called a curette to scrape away the wart, often after it's first anesthetized with a local anesthetic and burned with an electric needle.

Curettage can cause scarring and is used for only the most serious warts. And it may not even kill off the virus, which may still be lurking in the skin around the wart.

Zap warts away. In laser surgery, the doctor gives you local anesthesia and uses a laser beam—frequently the carbon dioxide (CO_2) laser—to destroy your wart. This method can successfully remove large, stubborn warts, but it causes scarring perhaps more than other treatments and requires a lot of follow-up care. It's also expensive, so you should probably try other treatments first.

Go for the works. Some doctors opt for combination treatments, like applying salicylic acid at night and in the morning, paring down the wart and applying another medication like Condylox, an alcohol solution that is technically approved only to treat genital warts.

Warding Off Warts

Although there's no foolproof way to avoid warts, you can do things to make your lovely skin a less hospitable host to these unsightly visitors.

Don't go barefoot. Never walk barefoot, especially at your health club or gym.

Keep your feet dry. "By reducing moisture, you reduce the environment the virus thrives in," says Dr. Gastwirth. If your feet tend to sweat, use foot powder; change your socks or stockings regularly, buy shoes in breathable materials (like leather and canvas, not vinyl) and let them dry out thoroughly between wearings.

Grab a clean towel. Don't share towels with other people. And if you already have warts, don't reuse a towel without washing it—you may reinfect yourself.

Be careful. If while you're trimming your nails you snip what turns out to be a wart, you'll spread the virus; if you nick a wart on your leg while shaving, you may end up spreading it everywhere that razor reaches.

CHAPTER TWENTY

Wrinkles

Erase Crinkles, Creases and Sleep Lines

Call them what you will—laugh lines, smile lines, crow's-feet or whatever euphemism you prefer. Wrinkles by any other name still top the list of skin-care worries. Ironic, considering that worrying about wrinkles only gives you more wrinkles.

The good news: If you're vigilant about protecting your skin, you don't have to get age-related wrinkles until relatively late in life. Plus, you can actually prevent most premature wrinkling.

So relax—there is something to smile about after all. You can stop the clock, or at least hit the snooze button, figuratively speaking, by stopping wrinkle-causing habits—and you can beat the clock altogether with the latest medical techniques for wrinkle removal.

Five Kinds of Wrinkles and How to Prevent Them

According to Melvin L. Elson, M.D., medical director of the Dermatology Center in Nashville and co-author of *The Good Look Book*, there are five distinct and identifiable causes of wrinkles—what he calls the five factors of the aging face. Other doctors concur.

Sun-dried wrinkles. The sun is the primary cause of extrinsic, or environmental, aging, damaging not just your complexion but the deepest layers of your skin, the dermis.

"The outer layer of your skin thickens to protect itself from the sun. This shell of dead surface skin causes the leathery look associated with sun damage," says Karen E. Burke, M.D., Ph.D., an attending physician at Cabrini Medical Center in New York City and adjunct clinical member of the Scripps Clinic and Research Foundation in California. The sun also hurts the dermis, destroying collagen and elastin, the materials that give skin its youthful tautness and elasticity.

You can get sun-induced crinkles as early as your teens, says Dr. Elson, which will turn into fine surface lines and dryness in your twenties. Beginning in your thirties, you might start to notice little freckle-like brown patches that are actually age spots. By your forties and fifties, skin can yellow and its fine lines become more prominent. "You may even get blackheads—one manifestation of sun damage—as your pores enlarge and clog," says Dr. Elson.

Fortunately, "the single most effective way to prevent wrinkles is to protect your skin from the sun," says Dr. Burke. And since it's never too late to start practicing "safe sun," begin slathering on a strong sunscreen with the same diligence you now apply moisturizer. Use sunscreen daily (rain or shine, since the sun's rays can penetrate cloud cover) wherever you are, whether you're at the beach or on the tennis court or simply walking to work, eating lunch outdoors or taking an afternoon jog.

The thin, delicate skin around your eyes is especially affected by the sun, so the sunscreen you daub under your eyes is more valuable than the priciest eye cream.

Old wrinkles. If it weren't for most environmental factors, like sun damage, you wouldn't get wrinkles until you were around 65 or 70, says Dr. Elson.

"Your skin doesn't age the way your heart or your kidneys do," says Albert M. Kligman, M.D., Ph.D. And aging skin doesn't lose as much collagen and elastin as you might think.

"After menopause, your skin produces a little less oil and gets a little thinner," says Dr. Kligman. "But by and large, the skin is a remarkable membrane."

To show just how remarkable, in the late 1980s Dr. Kligman and a team of researchers began studying the skin of Japanese monks, some in their nineties. Says Dr. Kligman, "They looked half their stated age. They never go out in the sun and their skin is marvelous, which shows that it's these external factors that ruin the skin."

Sleep lines. If you snooze on your side or stomach, your sleep habits can show up on your face as early as your midtwenties.

"Sleep lines" are easy to identify because they cut across ordinary wrinkles in a pattern that doesn't make sense—usually along the side of the chin or cheeks in women, according to Dr. Elson.

In your twenties, these lines disappear in a few hours. But if you don't stop sleeping on your face, by your forties and fifties, sleep lines will linger into your waking hours—"deep when you get up in the morning and deep when you go to bed at night," says Dr. Elson.

You can prevent sleep lines by teaching yourself to sleep on your back. Placing a firm pillow or two under your knees will help you stay in position until you drop off to sleep.

Expression lines. Horizontal lines across the forehead, vertical frown lines between the eyebrows and laugh lines at the sides of the mouth are caused by years of repetitive but unavoidable facial expressions like blinking and eating—even kissing. Expression lines can make their debut as faint lines around age 20, deepening as you

Face-Lift Alternatives:
Do You Really Want to Give Yourself a Lift?

Before you commit to getting collagen injections, a peel or Retin-A treatment, it's important that you know exactly what the results will be.

While the media often refer to these wrinkle-removing methods as face-lift alternatives or face-lifts without surgery, both terms are wrong: Only a face-lift can redrape loose, sagging skin. Collagen, peels and Retin-A treatment only remove lines and wrinkles and will not tighten bags and sags at all.

And while it doesn't involve an incision, the deep phenol peel—one of the most drastic wrinkle treatments—is actually a form of surgery.

"Surgery is an invasive procedure that changes the skin in a way that requires it to heal," says Melvin L. Elson, M.D., medical director of the Dermatology Center in Nashville and co-author of *The Good Look Book*. "Burning the skin—the action of a peel—does exactly that."

hit your thirties and forties. Lip lines (tiny vertical lines above the upper lip) may make their debut in your thirties but can appear much earlier if you smoke.

To help you stop the unnecessary grimacing that leads to wrinkles, look into a hand mirror while you're talking on the phone and watch for excessive lip pursing, nose wrinkling and grimacing, suggests Dr. Burke. Then, stick tape wherever you see expression lines talking hold—across your forehead, between your eyebrows, at the corners of your lips—and for a few minutes, practice talking without disturbing the tape. "Lucky people can even learn to smile without wrinkling their eyes," says Dr. Burke.

Squinting repeatedly causes crow's-feet—another type of expression line—along the corners of your eyes. Dark sunglasses are your first line of defense against crow's-feet, so wear them when you're outdoors. If you're squinting indoors, you may need corrective lenses or a stronger prescription if you already wear them. Also, don't read in dim light, and stop when your eyes are tired.

Gravity-prone grooves. The first areas of your face to show the effects of gravity (usually in your midthirties) are the corners of the mouth and the eyelids. In your forties, the nose-to-mouth lines that began as expression lines become creases, then actual folds. As you head into your fifties, gravity eventually affects the jawline and chin—and even the tip of the nose and the ears, which actually lengthen.

While you may be able to improve superficial wrinkles with various treatments, "only cosmetic surgery can undo deeper creases caused by gravity," says Dr. Elson.

Draw the Line at Skin-Wrinkling Habits

If there's been one breakthrough in wrinkle research over the years, it's been this: You have far more control over wrinkles than anyone ever dreamed. Here's how to avoid premature wrinkles.

Stub out the butts. Only the sun damages skin more than smoking. Heavy smokers are nearly five times more likely to show premature wrinkling than nonsmokers, according to research by Donald P. Kadunce, M.D., at the University of Utah Health Sciences Center in Salt Lake City. If you smoke and sunbathe, you'll wrinkle even more.

Squinting through cigarette smoke deepens lines around the eyes, and repeated puffing etches deep lines around the lips and may hollow the cheeks. Smokers also find themselves with gray and leathery complexions because their skin doesn't get enough oxygen—nicotine strangles the small blood vessels in the face.

If you think you can simply have a face-lift to repair the smoke damage, think again. "Most doctors won't perform de-aging procedures like collagen injections, face-lifts or deep peels on smokers," says Dr. Elson. "Smokers bruise more easily than nonsmokers and risk other side effects from surgery that nonsmokers don't." So you'll most likely have to stop smoking before a dermatologist will treat your lines or wrinkles.

Dump the yo-yo dieting. Gaining and losing the same 20 pounds is tough on your skin as well as your morale. Over time, the skin on your face may stretch until it won't snap back. The result: increased sagging. Maintaining your ideal weight by exercising more and practicing moderation in how much you eat will not only help keep your skin youthfully firm but also promote a healthy glow.

Forget facial aerobics. No matter what you may have read elsewhere, you can't grimace your way to tauter skin. Facial exercises have long been controversial, but leading medical experts firmly believe that facial contortions don't keep wrinkles at bay. "In fact, most of these exercises can accentuate wrinkles, because they use the very facial muscles that cause wrinkles," says Dr. Burke.

Experts also advise that you stay away from electrical gadgets like facial vacuum cleaners, so-called facial irons that are warmed up and applied to the face, and any other devices designed to manipulate the skin.

"You should treat your skin very tenderly and lovingly," says Dr. Elson. "It's a living thing and replaces itself every 28 days. If you mess up its cycle, it's really difficult to get it back in tune."

Don't be a skin guinea pig. The best skin-care strategy is "less is more." "Women tend to do too much rather than too little to their skin, and the problem isn't with lipsticks and blushers but skin-care products," says Dr. Kligman. So don't be too quick to try exotic skin-care products in the hope of staving off wrinkles; you may end up hurting your skin rather than helping it.

Decreasing the Damage

If you already have wrinkles, most experts doubt that over-the-counter creams will help. But don't fret: You do have several wrinkle-fighting options to choose from. Here are some treatments the experts say work.

Buff lines away. If you have fine wrinkles, mild exfoliation will slough off the dry top layer of your skin so it appears smoother. "The tiny wrinkles around the mouth and eyes are particularly likely to respond," says Dr. Burke. She recommends using a slightly abrasive facial sponge like a Buf Puf, available in any drugstore's skin-care section. "The rubbing action should be done perpendicular to the direction of the wrinkle," Dr. Burke explains. "Buff a little with a moist pad and your cleanser every night. But you can overdo it, so use restraint and common sense." Let your skin be your guide; buffing it once a week might be enough, advises Dr. Kligman. "And because exfoliating removes some of your skin's protective outer layer, it's even more important to use a sunscreen," says Dr. Burke.

Caution: Don't try exfoliation if you have fair or sensitive skin or if your complexion is prone to dilated blood vessels. And don't exfoliate your face with grainy scrubs, either. They're too harsh and can irritate your skin and eyes.

Try alpha hydroxy acids. Alpha hydroxy acids (AHAs) are mild acids derived from natural ingredients that appear to reduce the appearance of fine lines and leave skin looking smoother, fresher and brighter. Many over-the-counter moisturizers and wrinkle creams now contain AHAs: Glycolic acid, derived from fruit, and lactic acid, derived from milk, are particularly popular.

Glycolic acid treatments, available in drugstores and skin-care salons, will give your skin "slow improvement over time," says Dr. Elson. But over-the-counter glycolic acid preparations aren't as strong as those a dermatologist can prescribe. More significantly, using glycolic acid products can enhance the effectiveness of a prescription product like Retin-A (topical tretinoin).

Doctor's-Office Wrinkle Remedies

Dermatologists and cosmetic surgeons can dramatically reduce wrinkles and renew your skin with numerous treatments. Just bear in mind that while these procedures may eliminate wrinkles, they won't reduce sagging. And because of certain risks and side effects, they may or may not be appropriate for you. Read on.

Hold the lines with Retin-A. Barring surgery, the best wrinkle treatment medical science has to offer is Retin-A (topical tretinoin), a cream-based derivative of vitamin A that's rubbed into the skin.

Dr. Kligman originally developed Retin-A to treat acne. Its skin-rejuvenating qualities came as a surprise: Retin-A reduces fine wrinkles and mottled pigmentation on the skin's surface and stimulates cell turnover, collagen production and blood flow in the dermis. Dermatologists also pretreat skin with Retin-A to maximize the effects of other rejuvenating treatments, like facial peels and dermabrasion. These in-office procedures are discussed below.

Generally speaking, you apply Retin-A (available only by prescription) every night for six months, then cut down to once or twice a week to maintain the cream's benefits. Retin-A may cause side effects like redness and flaking; it also causes extreme photosensitivity. But you can usually minimize these side effects by using a moisturizer with added sunscreen in the morning and by avoiding the sun.

A freshening face peel. Using a variety of acid solutions, dermatologists can actually peel away damaged layers of skin to reveal the new, fresh skin beneath.

Depending on the type of acid used, facial peels can be light, medium or deep. For a light peel, dermatologists frequently use glycolic acid. A stronger chemical acid called trichloroacetic acid (TCA) is used for medium peels, while phenol—an extremely strong acid—is reserved for serious wrinkling.

The deeper the peel, the harder it is on your skin and the longer it takes for skin to recover. You'll look presentable right after a very light glycolic acid peel, but if you opt for a deep phenol peel, you'll need weeks to recover from scabbing and redness before your new skin is ready to face the world.

Filler injections. An experienced dermatologist can plump out creases and folds with a variety of substances, from collagen to your own fat. The down side, however, is that the effects of filler injections usually don't last very long because your body eventually absorbs the filler material. So you'll most likely have to repeat the procedure.

Dermabrasion. To perform this exfoliation technique, dermatologists use a rotating wire brush to remove damaged skin. As with a deep peel, it takes weeks to recover from the procedure.

Even Newer Ways to Doctor Up Wrinkles

Doctors are refining and even combining these techniques for even better results. The buff peel, invented by David Harris, M.D., a California dermatologist, is especially effective on fine lines around the eyes and above the upper lip caused by sun damage. The technique is a two-step process: Skin is first buffed with a special type of sandpaper, then treated with a medium-depth TCA peel. The buffing

A Guide to Treatment Options for Wrinkles

Not all wrinkles are alike, so treatment depends on what kind you have and where they show up. Here's an overview of various wrinkle treatments often offered by dermatologists.

If You Have	The Cause May Be	Your Dermatologist May Suggest
Fine facial wrinkles, crow's-feet at corners of eyes, whistle lines at corners of lips	→ Sun damage → Smoking → Age	→ Using a sunscreen with a high sun protection factor (SPF) → Quitting smoking → Exfoliation once a week (especially for crow's-feet and whistle lines) → Glycolic acid products → Retin-A treatment → Glycolic acid or trichloroacetic acid (TCA) peel → Retin-A and liquid nitrogen → Dermabrasion
Horizontal lines across forehead, vertical lines between eyebrows, laugh lines at corners of mouth, nose-to-mouth folds, drooping eyelids, sagging skin	→ Unavoidable facial movements (blinking, smiling, frowning) → Yo-yo dieting → Age	→ Sleeping on your back, placing a pillow under your knees to keep you in position → Maintaining a desirable weight → Filler injections (for nose-to-mouth folds) → Cosmetic surgery (face-lift, eye-lift)
Deep wrinkles	→ Premature sun damage → Age	→ Dermabrasion → Deep phenol peel

helps the TCA penetrate more deeply into the skin. Performed under light sedation, the procedure takes about 90 minutes, and results may last up to ten years, according to Dr. Harris.

Another one-two punch: Retin-A and liquid nitrogen. Dr. Burke developed this 60- to 90-minute facial treatment, in which skin is first treated with Retin-A, which is applied under a medical heating lamp to increase its penetration. The liquid nitrogen is then used to quicken cell turnover and peel dry, surface skin. Dr. Burke recommends you undergo the treatments every two weeks for four months, then about one a month for a year. You start seeing results after three or four treatments, says Dr. Burke.

The Dermappraisal: Customized Crinkle Relief

To celebrate your birthday, you've decided to give yourself a present—a day of line smoothing by a dermatologist. The only problem is, you're not sure which treatment will put your best face forward.

To find out, ask for a professional dermappraisal—a skin exam that analyzes your skin's individual aging process and outlines a line-by-line treatment plan.

What kind of wrinkles you have—and how you acquired them—will determine the best course of action. Say you have the beginnings of sun damage—fine facial lines, a few age spots, but no deep wrinkles or folds. Your dermappraisal might show that at-home skin care, rather than in-office treatment, would best address your skin's needs. Dr. Elson's sun-damage repair kit includes using Retin-A, sunscreens and glycolic acid products—in concentrations tailored to your skin's particular needs. If you want, you can also get an in-office peel. How strong a peel depends on the condition of your skin.

Or maybe you have deep nose-to-mouth folds, a few frown lines, some fine lines and crow's-feet and a yellowed complexion. This kind of wrinkling may call for at-home skin care to undo fine lines and discoloration, followed by in-office collagen injections to treat the folds and frown lines. Or if getting older has hollowed out your cheeks, a dermatologist might replace lost fat with fat transplants or implants.

See also the chapters on moisturizers (chapter 27), sunscreen (chapter 28), wrinkle creams (chapter 29), chemical peels (chapter 45), collagen injections and other filler techniques (chapter 46), dermabrasion (chapter 48) and Retin-A (chapter 51).

PART TWO

A Guide to Cosmetics
and
Skin-Care Products

CHAPTER TWENTY-ONE

Bath and After-Bath Treatments

Sensuous (and Sensible) Skin Soothers

Are you pouring capful after capful of bath oil into the tub, wondering why your dry, flaky skin just isn't responding?

According to many dermatologists, you might as well be pouring most bath oils right down the drain! Why? Because, as the saying goes, oil and water don't mix.

That's not to say you shouldn't use bath oil, or any number of other terrific bath and after-bath products. You just need to know how to use them correctly.

The Bath-Treatment Basic

The condition of your skin will tell you whether you need to use no-nonsense bath treatments to soothe dry skin or more pampering products to satisfy your body and soul.

But before the bubbles, the buffing: To renew your skin all over, many women enjoy using a loofah (a rough-textured mitt or sponge that removes dead skin cells), says Cheryl Renella, owner of Channing's Day Spa in Chicago. But these rough and nubbly skin scrubbers never seem to dry out, especially in high-humidity areas like the bathroom, and lingering moisture helps bacteria breed. So if you want to polish your skin, it's safer to use an exfoliant. These grainy scrubs slough off dead skin, leaving you glowing from head to toe.

Many exfoliants are formulated with finely ground nuts and nut shells. There are lots of exfoliants on the market, formulated with both natural and man-made granules; one of Channing's specialty products is a body scrub made with ground loofah, oatmeal and almonds.

Exfoliate with your fingers or a washcloth in a vigorous circular massage motion. By the way, a plain washcloth paired with any cleanser becomes a gentle exfoliator when you use this motion.

But don't scrub too hard: Exfoliants may irritate your skin. And if you have dry or sensitive skin, avoid these products altogether. Keep in mind that exfoliants should not be used on facial skin—it's too delicate for harsh scrubbing.

Beauty and the Bath: Mixing Business and Pleasure

Only a few years ago, you had to go to a beauty spa for body treatments. Now you can have your hydrotherapy at home: Just fill your tub, pick your product (anything from Dead Sea salts to Egyptian mud) and hop in.

In fact, we're all in a lather over bath products. Entire stores devoted to skin- and body-care products are cropping up all over the country. Goodebodies, The Body Shop, H_2O Plus and Bath & Body Works are among the best-known national chains. And more and more local skin-care salons and day spas (salons that offer the body-conditioning treatments that used to be available only at health spa resorts) are launching their own bath-product lines.

This explosion of bubbles, salts, gels, foams and lotions, scented with everything from flowers to fruit, adds to the pleasure principle of bathing. These products are best suited for women with normal skin, however; they aren't really skin-treatment products per se. But when familiar names in facial skin care launch bath products, you get the best of both worlds: safe, effective cleansing in a pleasurable format.

For the sensuous showerer, gels may be the bath extravagance of choice. "If you want to pamper yourself, gels bring out fragrance in a much nicer way than soaps," says Sven Thormahlen, Ph.D., director of product development at Beiersdorf, makers of Nivea, Eucerin and Aquaphor. Bath junkies may want to try another effective, yet pleasurable, skin treatment: VitaSpa, from the makers of VitaBath, one of the original bath treatments. VitaSpa is actually an assortment of bath and after-bath products that combine skin conditioning with a fresh, invigorating fragrance.

Bathing Dry Skin: Easy Does It

No matter how much you love to soak, overbathing can be too much of a good thing. Even if you use gentle cleansing products, taking too many long baths, just like overcleansing your face, can hurt rather than help your skin.

To calm fussy skin, limit baths to ten minutes. Also, bathe in warm rather than hot water to keep from stripping away your skin's own protective oils, says Rodney S. W. Basler, M.D., head of a task force on sports medicine and assistant professor of dermatology at the University of Nebraska Medical Center in Omaha.

And be sure to choose a mild cleansing product. Harsh soaps, typically deodorant soaps, can cause irritation if you have dry, sensitive

Kitchen-Cabinet Skin Soothers

Fluffy bubbles and exotic scents can turn a bath into a sensual experience. But if you want a good old-fashioned treatment for dry skin, look no further than your pantry.

Plain oatmeal is a time-honored remedy that calms dryness by leaving a film on your skin that seals in water. Think of it as an invisible shield to fend off irritation and the urge to scratch. Plus, oatmeal is easy to use. Simply fill an old nylon stocking with dry oatmeal, tie up the little bundle and throw it in the tub. To get the film without the fuss, use a fine-milled oatmeal product like Aveeno.

Baking soda, another home remedy for dry skin, sometimes relieves itching triggered by contact with water.

"No one knows exactly why baking soda works," says Stephen M. Purcell, D.O., chairman of the Division of Dermatology at the Philadelphia College of Osteopathic Medicine. Some experts think baking soda might change water's ion content so that less is absorbed into the skin's outer layer.

For Sensitive Skin:
Making Sense of Scented Products

" 'Fragrance-free' is a popular sales pitch," says Albert M. Kligman, M.D., Ph.D. "Perhaps too much has been made of it."

In fact, only 1 to 3 percent of the population may be allergic to certain ingredients in cosmetics, most commonly fragrances and preservatives.

What's more, it might not even be the fragrance that's to blame. If you're using a bubble bath, the detergents that create those bubbles might be irritating your skin.

If you simply need a mild cleanser, try Oil of Olay's Bath Bar or a detergent-based liquid cleanser, suggests Dr. Kligman. "Both Lever Brothers and Procter & Gamble have good brands," he adds. A very mild no-soap cleanser, like Eucerin or Cetaphil, may soothe sensitive, extremely dry skin.

If you do have allergic skin, try the Basis brand of cleansers, which are both fragrance- and preservative-free; the Basis bar is also superfatted to prevent dryness.

skin or a chronic skin problem, says Albert M. Kligman, M.D., Ph.D.

"Even people with normal skin can develop eczema if they shower more than once a day with a harsh deodorant soap that strips oil from the skin," adds Dr. Basler. "Shower in the morning, then shower after a gym workout using deodorant soap—do this twice a day and after two weeks, you'll end up with xerotic (dry-skin) eczema or even nummular eczema." Nummular eczema is particularly unpleasant—coin-shaped patches that blister and ooze.

Dermatologists often recommend body bars like Dove, Tone and Caress rather than deodorant soaps. If you're concerned about body odor, though, use a regular deodorant or use a deodorant soap in strategic locations only. To further avoid serious dry-skin conditions, shake off excess water as soon as you get out of the tub and pat yourself dry, then immediately lock in the moisture you've absorbed with a super-rich emollient (see below).

After-Bath Moisture Boosters

If you have normal skin, using lotions after bathing is fine. You might choose a lotion that's part of the same line as your bath cleanser, especially if you use scented products and want the depth of fragrance that "layering" products can provide.

But if your skin is more than just slightly dry, slathering on a lotion probably isn't enough. "People use lotions because they're easy and convenient, but many are mostly alcohol and water," explains Jon M. Hanifin, M.D., professor of dermatology at Oregon Health Sciences University in Portland. Here's how to hydrate right.

Soak first, then add oil. Bath or body oils come in hundreds of formulations. There's plain old baby oil, exotic scented oils, oils you pour—even oils you spray.

But most of these products are only marginally effective, says Dr. Kligman, especially if you're pouring them in before you step into the tub. Why? Because if you put the oil in the tub before you get in, a surface of oil will form over your skin, actually preventing water from hydrating it!

To get your bath oil's maximum moisturizing benefits, soak in plain water for a few minutes. Then pour in your oil. When you get out, a film of oil will form on your skin and trap the water that has soaked in.

For even better results, apply oil after you get out of the tub. "Put it on right out of the container—the dose is 100 times better," says Dr. Kligman. "It's also safer; oil in the tub can be very slippery."

Moisture-rich creams and ointments. Seriously dry skin needs a richer emollient to lock in the water it has absorbed. If the emollient isn't heavy enough, your skin can feel drier than ever once the water evaporates.

Dr. Hanifin suggests a heavy-duty cream, "something that doesn't pour!" he says. Petroleum jelly rates high on the lists of many doctors. So do products like Eucerin, available in a cream or lotion, which doesn't have the thin consistency of traditional lotions, and Aquaphor, an ointment. Bath products formulated with lanolin can also be effective on dry skin, says Dr. Kligman. Some dermatologists say lanolin is an important sensitizer, however. So don't use moisturizers formulated with lanolin if you know you have sensitive skin.

See also the chapter on eczema (chapter 10).

CHAPTER TWENTY-TWO

Cleansers

Lose the Grime, Keep the Glow

*I*t's 11:00 P.M. and you're staring bleary-eyed into the bathroom mirror, trying to see if any trace of the day's makeup is left on your face.

It looks pretty clean. So do you really have to cleanse?

Much as you'd like to just slip into bed, you owe it to your face to spend two or three minutes (yes, that's all it should take) cleaning up your act. Along with the barely visible vestiges of your morning makeup is a fair amount of grime—pollution, smoke, exhaust fumes—not to mention dead cells begging to be sloughed off. A thorough cleansing with the right product gets rid of this pore-clogging, skin-dulling dirt. Your morning reward: fresh, radiant skin.

The Real Dirt on Cleansers

Cleansers are formulated with one of three basic ingredients: soap, synthetic detergents or oil. You'll also find them in many formats, like bars, foamy liquids, milky lotions and creams.

While you'll want to pick a product that suits your individual skin type, how well a cleanser rinses away is important, too, says Mitchell S. Wortzman, Ph.D., president of Neutrogena Dermatologics in Los Angeles. Why? Because a cleanser can irritate your

An Easy Cleanser Test

Is your cleanser doing its job—or doing it too well? To find out, take this tightness test: Your cleanser should make your skin feel faintly taut right after you use it.

This slight tightness will tell you the cleanser has removed the surface oils that collect dirt, explains Mitchell S. Wortzman, Ph.D., president of Neutrogena Dermatologics in Los Angeles. But if the tautness lasts more than 10 to 15 minutes, switch to a gentler, milder cleanser.

If your face still feels tight even after you've applied your moisturizer, you could have irritable skin, says Dr. Wortzman, and may need to see a dermatologist.

skin if it leaves a sticky residue behind. So the faster your cleanser goes down the drain, the less it can damage your skin. "Think of it this way: the easier a cleanser washes off, the milder it is," says Dr. Wortzman.

Your cleanser should also leave your skin ready for moisturizer, unless your skin is so naturally oily you don't need one. Yet you shouldn't count on a moisturizer to compensate for a harsh cleanser. Even a mild product can aggravate your skin if you use it too often.

Clean-Up Acts

Your choice of cleanser often comes down to whether you like the feel of a bar, the foam of a liquid or the slickness of a cream. Luckily, you'll likely be able to match your favorite cleansing format with your skin type. Here's a list of your wash-up options.

True soap. True soap, which comes in liquid and bar form, often has a base of coconut oil, tallow or other fatty acids. While true soap is generally thought to be the harshest on the skin, liquid soaps are usually milder than soap bars because their stripping action is diluted by water and other ingredients.

You might not want to use any soap—either true or soap-free (see below)—if you live in a hard-water area. Minerals in hard water can leave a filmy residue on your skin.

Soap-free cleansers. These nonsoaps, either bar or liquid, have a detergent base. The cosmetics industry calls these products syndets—short for synthetic detergents. But don't shy away from the *D* word: Detergents can be milder than true soaps. In fact, superfatted soaps, which contain added emollients like olive oil or cocoa butter, are also soap-free and are often called beauty bars.

If you want to make sure you're getting a syndet, check the product's label for the words *soap-free* or *nonsoap*.

Liquid cleansers. You'll generally find these products in two basic formulations: clear, foaming gels for oilier skin and stroke on/tissue- or wash-off milky lotions for dry or delicate skin. Because they foam or lather more than other cleansers, they usually

A Super Skin-Care Routine

Heavy makeup, hot camera lights . . . how does an actress manage to get her skin clean after she wraps for the day?

Ask Tracy Scoggins (*Lois & Clark: The New Adventures of Superman*), who manages to keep her skin flawless without a complicated or expensive skin-care regimen. Here's her tried-and-true routine.

"First, I rub petroleum jelly all around my eyes—lids, lashes and all," says Tracy. "Then, using my fingers or a clean washcloth, I wash my face with a soap called Oilatum (an inexpensive soap formulated for normal to dry skin). The soap takes off my eye makeup, but it's not as harsh on the areas I've soaked with petroleum jelly."

After she finishes cleansing, Tracy moisturizes her face with Complex-15, the same product she's been using for years. "I put it on right after cleansing, while my face is still damp," she says.

Twice a week, Tracy buffs away dead skin cells with a facial scrub. (While many dermatologists discourage the use of these scrubs, they're extremely popular.) And that's it.

rinse away better, too, which cuts the risk of their leaving an irritating residue on your skin.

Cleansing creams. These cleansers, which you rinse away with warm water, remove with a wet washcloth or simply tissue off, rely primarily on mineral oil to remove makeup and dirt. Their cleansing action is based on the idea that like dissolves like—the oil in the cream lifts off the oil, grime and makeup on your face. But, needless to say, they don't rinse away as well as other cleansers.

Choosing a Cleanser

Let's face it: Many of us pick a cleanser based more on its packaging or ad hype than its effect on our skin. Others believe that only plain soap and water get skin really clean.

To keep your skin glowing, you'll need to change your thinking, because what you don't know can hurt your skin. Using a too-strong cleanser when you don't need it can parch your skin, making fine lines more noticeable or even irritating your skin. By the same token, using a cleanser that's too oily for your skin can lead to breakouts.

Fortunately, many skin-care companies make cleansers for normal skin, dry skin, combination skin, sensitive skin and so on. So it's simple to match up your face with the cleanser that suits it.

Cleansing oily skin. An oily complexion needs and can tolerate a stronger cleanser because it's a magnet for dirt and environmental pollutants, explains James N. Bollinger, Ph.D., associate director of pharmaceutical research and development at Galderma Laboratories in Fort Worth, Texas.

But consider steering clear of a true soap: It can strip even oily skin of its natural protection as it lathers away dirt. Better to try a liquid cleanser formulated for oily skin. One example is Pond's Foaming Cleanser & Toner In One.

Gentle cleansing for dry skin. The drier your skin, the creamier your cleanser should be, so opt for a tissue-off cleansing cream or a lighter cleansing lotion. For very dry or sensitive skin, a totally detergent-free tissue-off cleanser is safest. You can also rinse off these cleansers or remove them with a soft, wet washcloth. Cleansing creams leave behind a moisturizing film, so if your skin is normal to slightly dry, you shouldn't need to use a separate moisturizer.

Needless to say, what you don't want on your face is soap. "Use the wrong soap for two weeks and I can guarantee that you'll notice wrinkles more," says Albert M. Kligman, M.D., Ph.D.

What's the wrong soap? It's sometimes hard to say: Soap isn't considered a cosmetic, so it's not required to carry an ingredients label. But you can cut your chances of choosing a true-soap product by avoiding any cleanser that lists sodium cocoate or sodium tallowate on its label.

Combination skin. You can probably use a cleanser formulated for normal or oily skin if you're shiny across your forehead, nose and chin (known as the T-zone). But if you want your very own cleanser, try a cleanser made specifically for combination skin. Neutrogena's Fresh Foaming Cleanser is only one of many; the no-soap formula balances T-zone oiliness with your skin's drier areas.

Sensitive skin. Cetaphil, which can be tissued or rinsed off, is the gold-standard soap-free cleanser dermatologists often recommend for very sensitive skin. If you have allergic skin, try gentle, fragrance- and preservative-free soapless cleansers like Basis, a bar, or Neutrogena Cleansing Wash, a liquid.

Try a liquid cleanser made for dry or sensitive skin, too. Says Dr. Kligman, "Some companies have introduced extremely mild liquid cleansers which are good for people who have sensitive or dry skin, eczema and rosacea."

Dr. Kligman has tested two liquid cleansers on people with sensitive skin: Oil of Olay Sensitive Skin Foaming Face Wash and Dove Liquid Beauty Wash. "I try to make their skin worse. If I don't, then I know I have a good cleanser," he says. And if they're gentle on delicate skin, they'll work on virtually every skin type.

The Top Five Cleansing Errors and How to Avoid Them

Is your cleansing regimen keeping your skin from looking its glowing best? Try quitting these five common cleansing gaffes.

Cleansing too often. Bad for dry skin, but bad for oily skin, too. Overwashing your face can stimulate your oil glands, making your skin even slicker. So no matter what your skin type, cleanse no more than twice a day with a cleanser formulated for your skin type.

Using too much cleanser. The less concentrated your cleanser, the gentler it is on your skin. So dilute a dot of liquid cleanser with water or lather up your bar in the palm of your hand before you suds up.

Using cleansing products that are too harsh. You might like the tingly feeling an alcohol-based astringent provides, but using it every day can lead to tight, flaky skin. In fact, astringent is often overkill even for oily skin. So let your skin be your guide.

Using products too harshly. Yes, whiteheads are aggravating— but overscrubbing won't help. Avoid abrasive facial pads or grainy scrubs, advise most experts. You might end up with blotchy, flaky skin or even tiny broken capillaries.

Not rinsing enough. Most women don't rinse away their cleansers thoroughly enough. When you think you're done rinsing, splash your face three more times.

Eye Makeup: Easy-Off Tips

You know good eye-makeup removers dissolve mascara easily without making you tug at the delicate skin around your eyes. But which remover formula is best: oily or nonoily? It depends.

You may want to try a gentle cleanser first, especially if you have sensitive skin. Cetaphil, among the gentlest facial cleansers available, effectively removes even waterproof mascara. "It's a little more work, but it won't irritate your skin or your eyes," says Dr. Bollinger.

Oily removers have their pluses and minuses. They can seep into your eyes, which is not pleasant, particularly if you wear contact lenses. Always remove your lenses before you take off your eye makeup. Plus, says Laura Geller, makeup artist and owner of Laura Geller Make-Up Studios, a cosmetics store in New York City, "if you can't get rid of the oily residue, your makeup will slide off when you try to apply it."

Oil-free eye-makeup removers are less messy, but you may want to avoid them if you have sensitive skin. If your lids are prone to redness, itching and irritation (specifically eyelid dermatitis), it's wise to stick to an oily remover.

See also the chapter on allergic skin (chapter 43).

CHAPTER TWENTY-THREE

Concealers

Perfecting the Great Cover-Up

Ever spend 20 minutes dabbing at a pimple on your chin or dark circles under your eyes, trying to get your concealer to conceal? Then you know these so-called cover-ups can often call attention to the very flaws you're trying to hide.

Not anymore: Concealers aren't the ghostly, ghastly lighteners they used to be. You'll find more shades that actually match your skin tone. That means raccoon eyes—those awful milky-white half-moons caused by using a too-light concealer—are a thing of the past. You'll also find concealers in sheer, creamy or thick coverage that match your specific masking needs—everything from dark circles to scars.

One Shade Doesn't Fit All

It used to be a challenge to find a concealer beyond the traditional fair, medium and dark. But now, concealers are as shade-specific as foundations. For example, Prescriptives Camouflage Cream comes in 16 shades and Lydia O'Leary's Covermark Face Magic comes in 13. And many more cosmetic companies offer 4 or more shades.

Generally speaking, the right color concealer is one shade lighter than your skin tone, says Laura Geller, makeup artist and owner of Laura Geller Make-Up Studios in New York City.

"But try before you buy," she says. "You'll probably want to test more than one shade, especially if you're trying to cover undereye circles (see below)." And try to look at the concealer in daylight, if possible; you'll be able to see whether it's too light, too dark or just right.

It's especially important to match your cover-up to your complexion if you're using a heavy concealer. Thicker products tend to tattle with a noticeable line of demarcation, especially if you're spot-applying rather than using them over your entire face.

No More Telltale Circles

Dark circles are unsightly, annoying—and surprisingly easy to cover, once you find the right concealer.

The right product is usually the creamiest, because the skin under the eyes is often dry. "It's not a good idea to apply a hard stick concealer directly to the undereye area—the skin is much too delicate," says Geller. So before using a stick concealer, she suggests softening it up first with your fingertip.

"Concealers in a wand or pot are creamiest," says Geller. Creamy undereye concealers include Maybelline Revitalizing Concealer (formulated with built-in moisturizers), Estee Lauder Automatic Cream Concealer and Signature Cream Concealer. Brighten up—not whiten up—your dark circles with these easy step-by-step instructions.

Prep for your concealer. If the skin under your eyes is dry, pat on a light eye cream to keep your concealer from appearing cakey or thick.

Apply foundation. Foundation hides dark circles to some degree and helps concealer glide on more smoothly than concealer alone.

Measure out your concealer. Using your index finger, pat a dime-size dot of creamy concealer, or a pea-size dab if you're using a wand concealer, under each eye.

Start covering up. Dab the concealer from the inner corner of your eye outward, using your index finger to pat it into place. Use as little concealer as possible around your eyes; the product will sink into fine lines after a few hours.

Check your work. Stand back from the mirror. If you can still see dark circles, pat on a tiny bit more concealer.

Blend. Feather the edges of the concealer into your foundation, lifting off excess concealer with a sponge or cotton square.

Finish up with powder. Using a very small, narrow makeup brush, dust on translucent powder to set the concealer. But don't use too much powder—it will accentuate crow's-feet and eventually cake into lines.

Hiding the Zit from Hell

You don't have to stare grimly at the same mocking pimple every day for a week. Many blemish concealers camouflage blemishes while they battle acne-causing bacteria.

Try over-the-counter tinted acne medications like Clearasil or Exact Pimple & Acne Medicated Tinted Cream or concealers formulated with the chemical exfoliant (which sloughs off dead skin cells)

Watch Flaws Vanish with These Expert Tips

The next time you're trying to hide the evidence of a 3:00 A.M. bedtime or cover a nasty pimple, follow these tips. You'll conceal the evidence without a trace.

Make up before you cover up. Apply your face makeup before your concealer so you won't disturb it while you're applying your foundation or blusher.

Do your eyes first, too. It will keep wayward flecks of shadow or mascara from getting mired in your undereye concealer. Apply a medicated blemish concealer before your foundation, however.

Don't cover crow's-feet. You may end up accentuating rather than hiding fine lines. "The less makeup you wear around the outer corners of your eyes, the better," says New York makeup expert Pablo Manzoni. That goes for powder, too.

Repair the damage. When your concealer sinks into crow's-feet, reblend it into your foundation with your fingertip, the corner of a cosmetic sponge or a sponge-tipped applicator.

Pencil out your flaws. Stick or pencil concealers, made by Shiseido, Artistry, Dermablend, Covermark and others, hit the spot when you're on the go. To use them in the thin-skinned undereye area, stroke the product along your fingertip, then pat on the coverage.

salicylic acid, such as Clinique's Acne Control Formula and Cover Girl Clarifying Concealer. Salicylic acid sloughs away the dead skin cells, thereby helping to eliminate blemishes.

Unlike regular concealers, medicated blemish cover-ups generally work best if you dab them directly on the blemish first, rather than last. So be sure to read your concealer's application directions.

To best hide your blemish, use a special camouflage brush to apply the concealer only over the pimple itself. You can find these stiff, synthetic-hair brushes, similar to a lip brush, in cosmetics stores. Then feather the edges of the concealer with your fingertip or the edge of a cosmetic sponge.

Never use an undereye concealer on a blemish. "The oils it contains could aggravate the pimple," says Geller.

Fast Fixes for More Serious Flaws

You'll need a heavier concealer to cover broken capillaries, a birthmark or port-wine stain, a burn, a scar or a condition like vitiligo. Both Geller and New York makeup expert Pablo Manzoni give high marks to Clinique's Continuous Coverage, available in six shades. It's very thick—almost like a stage makeup—and will hide scars as well as other skin imperfections.

You might also try the pioneers of serious concealers, Covermark and Dermablend, both available in department stores. "These 'paramedical' products, formulated to cover severe skin problems, are made to cover large areas and are waterproof," says Geller.

Dermablend Cover Creme Foundation is formulated especially for the face and comes in eight shades. Dermablend Leg & Body Cover offers six shades.

Another concealer, Derma Color by Kryolan, is actually a stage makeup, available at theatrical supply stores. According to Geller, Derma Color hides imperfections from dark circles to scars.

Do not use tinted underbases for serious concealing jobs. Created to even out skin tone, these concealers supposedly correct sallowness, usually with a lilac shade, or ruddiness, with yellow or green. But they just don't work, according to many makeup pros. "You can look ghastly if you misuse them," says Manzoni.

The only exception to this rule is if you have rosacea (pronounced ro-ZAY-shuh), a skin condition with acne that can turn skin extremely ruddy. In this case, using an underbase tinted green will help conceal rosacea's redness.

CHAPTER TWENTY-FOUR

Eye Makeup

Looking Good without Looking "Done"

*E*ye makeup, like lipstick, is the candy of cosmetics. All those pretty colors, packaged in pretty jars, palettes, pencils and tubes, can be pretty irresistible.

But as alluring as these shadows, liners and mascaras may be, the secret of perfectly applied eye makeup is using as few products as possible and applying them with a light hand. Even a bare-bones application of eye makeup (a hint of shadow, a touch of liner and a light coat or two of mascara) will give your eyes an extra sparkle and light up your whole appearance.

This keep-it-simple approach to eye makeup makes it easy to use, too. So don't worry if you're all thumbs with an eye pencil or lash curler; a few quick lessons in technique will help you avoid the Tammy Faye look while enhancing your eyes' natural beauty. And by the way, even if you've been applying makeup with confidence for years and are happy with the results, it's a good idea to review this chapter and reevaluate your routine. Nothing adds unnecessary years to a woman's face like an outdated eye-makeup look.

Shadow Play

To turn standard-issue lids extraordinary, turn to eye shadow, which comes in a variety of powder, pencil and cream formats.

As with other cosmetics, however, you'll want to choose your eye shadow with your skin type in mind. De-emphasize dry skin by using creamy shadows, which will glide rather than drag across your lids. If your skin tends to be oily, choose powdered shadows, which are less likely to slip or streak if your face gets shiny.

Whatever your skin type, avoid frosted shadows; they're flattering on only a very few women, says Laura Geller, makeup artist and owner of Laura Geller Make-Up Studios, a cosmetics store in New York City. They can make your lids look crepelike and draw attention to bags and wrinkles. Worse, the tiny, shiny flecks that give iridescent shadows their sparkle can irritate your eyes, particularly if you wear contact lenses. So stick with matte (nonshiny) shades instead, advises Geller.

A Question of Color

While eye-shadow shades come and go, a good rule of thumb is to keep color low-key, not Las Vegas. But just as bad as shocking purple lids is matching your shadow to your outfit, says New York makeup expert Pablo Manzoni. "Thankfully, women are no longer told to match their eye shadow to what they're wearing," he says.

Instead, match your shadow to your skin tone, says Geller. "The lighter your skin, the lighter the shade should be," she says. If you're a fair-skinned blonde, for instance, wear sea foam rather than hunter green; if you're an olive-skinned brunette, you can carry a stronger shade.

Or you could simplify the whole color conundrum and stick to neutrals, says Geller. Neutrals include the entire range of flesh tones from ebony to ivory, with grays, browns, peaches, coffees, sands and other earth tones in between. "Neutrals are very natural looking," says Geller. "It's almost impossible to use them incorrectly, and they accent your eyes subtly, yet expressively."

As you get older, you can still use a hint of color on your lids; it can give pale or sallow skin an instant lift. Just keep the shade subtle, says Geller—a gray shadow with blue undertones, for example, rather than bold blue shadow or a brown shadow with green undertones rather than a parrot green shade.

What not to use on mature lids: colors that are too dark—they'll make your lids appear sunken—and shades of pink. "They'll make your eyes look red and tired," says Geller.

Step-by-Step Shadow

The key to perfect eye shadow is in the blending; color looks more natural when you can't count the number of shades you've used.

Prep your lids. Dot your lids with foundation from lashline to eyebrow, then dust them with translucent powder. This base gives shadow something to cling to and helps color last longer.

Shadow your brow bone. Using a sponge-tipped applicator,

The Top Five Eye-Makeup Goofs and How to Avoid Them

As with blush, too much eye color in the wrong place can end up detracting from your appearance rather than enhancing your looks. Here's how to sidestep the biggest eye-makeup mishaps.

Maxed-out mascara. Stiff, clumpy lashes are less than alluring. So don't use more than two or three coats of mascara, and use an eyelash comb between applications.

Overdone eyeliner. Using too much eyeliner or not applying it neatly looks hard or—worse—tacky. "If you notice it, you're wearing too much," says Laura Geller, makeup artist and owner of Laura Geller Make-Up Studios, a cosmetics store in New York City.

Raccoon eyes. Using mascara on your lower lashes and lining your lower lids can accentuate bags, dark circles, lines and puffiness. Keep the focus on your upper lids.

Stretching delicate skin. Closing one eye or stretching your lids when you apply eyeliner or shadow can distort your makeup's appearance when you let go. "Look straight ahead with open eyes," advises New York makeup expert Pablo Manzoni.

Hurried application. Slapdash shadow, wandering liner, mascara that speckles your cheeks...yuck. Don't sell your look short. "Perfectly applied and blended makeup is the mark of a woman who's really pulled together," says Manzoni.

sweep a neutral shadow on your brow bone from the crease of your upper lid to your eyebrow line.

Here's where a bit of cosmetic trickery can work to your benefit: Light colors bring an area forward and dark shades make it recede. So use a brown, gray-brown or mocha shadow to push back a brow bone that is too prominent and a beige, peach or ivory to bring a recessive one forward. But always use a neutral shade on this area; shadowing your brow bone blue or green will draw attention to the color rather than your eyes.

Color your lids. Now sweep a contrasting color on your lids from the lashline to the crease. Apply the strongest concentration of color closest to your lashline. Then blend the lid and brow colors. "Color should fade out as it approaches the crease of your eyelids," says Geller.

Eyeliner: The Right Shade, in the Right Amount, in the Right Place

Although Cleopatra's extended-to-the-ears eyeliner was a little extreme, she understood its cosmetic value: Eyeliner shapes and enhances your eyes by making your lashes appear thicker.

While eyeliner comes in pencil, liquid and cake form (which requires a brush and water to apply), liquid eyeliners don't stretch or pull your lids like eye pencils can and are more convenient than cake eyeliner. If you prefer eye pencils, though, try eyeliner pens, which offer pencil-point precision in a flowing formula.

Lining up with color. "The color of your liner should be as deep as the color of your lashes and brows," says Geller. So if you're a fair-skinned blonde, steer clear of black, brown and navy liners and choose a rich violet or deep blue instead. And every woman—even blondes—can wear a deep khaki green, smoky gray or smoky blue.

Wobble-free lining tips. Can't draw a straight line? Don't worry; with practice, you'll straighten out your act. In the meantime, consider using eyeliner pencils, which are easier to control than liquid or cake liner. Or steady your shaky fingers by steadying your elbow on a flat surface and anchoring it firmly with your other hand. You can also cheat by applying liquid liner in dots along the roots of your lashes rather than trying for a thin, perfect line.

Whichever liner formula you choose, apply it as close to the roots of your lashes as you can. Says Geller, "Aim for a thin line, not a thick stripe, and use a cotton swab to soften a heavy application."

You can give your eyes added definition by lining your lower lids, but beware: undereye liner can emphasize dark circles, puffiness, bags and wrinkles.

Mascara: How to Plump Up the Volume

Most women have a love-hate relationship with mascara. It highlights your eyes by making your lashes look thicker and longer, but it flakes, globs and clumps. And then there's taking it off. To avoid such mascara disasters, try these lush-lash tips.

Choose a fiber-free mascara. Many mascaras use threadlike fibers that adhere to lashes to add length or thickness. "If you wear contact

Makeup Hygiene Prevents Nasty Eye Infections

A beautiful shade of shadow or a creamy pencil liner can give you gorgeous eyes—or an eye infection. So practicing good hygiene is an essential part of any eye-makeup routine.

→ Wash all your eye-makeup brushes once a week with an antiseptic liquid soap, says Laura Geller, makeup artist and owner of Laura Geller Make-Up Studios, a cosmetics store in New York City. Allow them to dry overnight, or use a blow-dryer.

→ Change the rubber pads on your eyelash curler every month.

→ Toss out mascara after three months. Remind yourself by dating tubes with write-on tape. Unopened mascara lasts indefinitely if you put it in the fridge, says Geller.

→ Sharpen eye pencils before you use them—every time. "A creamy pencil can harbor bacteria," says Geller.

→ To discourage contamination, keep powder shadows tightly shut between use.

→ When you're shopping, don't try on testers at cosmetics counters unless disposable applicators are provided.

lenses or if your eyes are sensitive, don't wear mascaras with added fibers," says Geller. "They tend to irritate your eyes. You may not feel it at first, but two hours later your eyes may start to burn."

Models swear by a fiber-free, beauty-industry standard: Maybelline's Great Lash. Other fiber-free formulas include Lash Out or Splash Out by L'Oreal and Max Factor's For Your Eyes Only Mascara, formulated especially for sensitive eyes.

Before you apply any mascara, though, wipe off the wand first to reduce the chance of clumping.

Stick to tried-and-true hues. Many of us have flirted with purple or green mascara but always come back to black—the best shade for lash definition, according to Geller. Generally speaking, though, mascara, like liner, should match the intensity of your lashes and brows. Geller suggests black mascara for brunettes and brown for blondes and redheads. To compliment gray hair, try navy, suggests Geller. "It will make the whites of your eyes look whiter and minimize redness if your eyes are tired," she says.

Black women who find that brown or black mascara disappears into their skin tone might try a purple or royal blue mascara, says Geller. "Both colors can give your eyes a little sparkle," she says.

Buy an eyelash curler. It may look like an instrument of torture, but an eyelash curler will make your lashes look lusher—and your eyes larger and brighter—than using mascara alone. And a lash curler isn't as hard to use as you might think.

To avoid losing precious lashes, curl them before you apply mascara and moisten them with a clear mascara or a drop of water to further reduce the chance of breakage. Then, with your eye open and looking downward, slip your upper lashes through the curler and squeeze. Hold for about five seconds. Don't pump the curler—it increases the risk of catching or pulling out your lashes.

Finally, apply a coat of mascara from lash root to tip. Then, while your lashes are still wet, declump them with a metal (not plastic) eyelash comb, available at beauty supply stores and drugstores.

If you can't fatten 'em, fake 'em. Perhaps your lashes have thinned as you've grown older—a natural occurrence, says Geller. If so, strip lashes can help camouflage a skimpy lashline. For the most natural-looking lashes, pick a soft brown; opt for black if you have very dark hair and coloring. You can trim them to the length and width you want, so choose fakes for thickness rather than length, says Geller. She also suggests using clear lash glue for the most natural look.

CHAPTER TWENTY-FIVE

Foundation, Blusher and Powder

Facing the World with a Youthful Glow

*W*hat's the difference between a magician performing a card trick and a woman applying her makeup?

Not much, when you consider just what a magical change makeup can make. Foundation can perk up a sallow complexion or tone down a ruddy one, give skin a smooth finish or minimize its imperfections. A light sweep of blusher lends your skin a healthy glow even if you're feeling a bit under the weather, while a dusting of powder sets other makeup, stops oily shine and even, in some cases, doubles as foundation. Given all these benefits, there's something downright enchanting about the way makeup can make us look—and feel.

If you're makeup-shy, however, you may be feeling downright dubious about all these cosmetic hosannas. But there are lots of good reasons to give makeup another chance. Today's products are lighter and sheerer than ever before, so you won't feel as if you're wearing a mask. Even better, one-shade-fits-all foundations and powders are a thing of the past. Complexion-specific products are now formulated with your skin in mind. And all you need to succeed in makeup wizardry is a few lessons on how to use your bag of tricks—cosmetics.

Base-ic Instinct: Picking the Perfect Foundation

Today's foundations, available in lots of formulas, including liquid, cream and cream-powder, do more than even out your skin tone or cover small imperfections. Many foundations actually protect with good-for-your-complexion extras like sunscreen or moisturizers. Says Sylvie Chantecaille, senior executive of creative marketing at Prescriptives in New York City, "Women now look at foundation as the most intelligent way to protect their skin."

Of course, the breathtaking assortment of foundations you'll find at the cosmetics counter can leave you blinking in bewilderment. But you can cut through the confusion by focusing on three basics: color, coverage and formulation.

No More Basic (Boring) Beige

What's the difference between honey and tawny beige, ivory and alabaster? If you don't know, don't fret: Matching a foundation to your skin tone can be simple, once you've mastered a few basics.

First, don't test a foundation's color on the back of your hand—a common mistake, says New York makeup expert Pablo Manzoni. "Try a foundation on your jawline so you'll see how it relates to your whole face—to your cheeks as well as your neck," he says.

You'll also need to determine your skin's undertone. No matter what your complexion—ruddy or olive, fair or ebony—your skin is either more sallow (yellow) or more ruddy (red), says Laura Geller, makeup artist and owner of Laura Geller Make-Up Studios, a cosmetics store in New York City.

"Determine whether your skin is more red or more yellow," advises Geller. "If you're ruddy, wear a foundation with some yellow to it to warm up your skin. If you're more sallow, cool down your warm tones with a rosier foundation." Very fair skin needs a foundation that looks more ivory than yellow, like alabaster, says Geller.

Black skin can be harder to match, says Geller. It's getting easier, though. While the Flori Roberts and Fashion Fair cosmetic lines are made specifically for black skin, other major cosmetic companies have also begun making foundations for black women.

If you have very black skin, compliment your blue-red undertone with a foundation that contains a good amount of red, says Geller. Lighter-skinned black women, whose complexions tend to be sallow, look best in bronzy or golden foundations.

Once you've found the perfect shade, you may decide to use less of it. "You can use foundation just where you need it, like your T-zone or the apples of your cheeks, to even out your skin tone," she says. Don't worry about looking spotty. If the foundation's consistency is sheer enough, you won't see makeup—just perfect skin.

Is Your Foundation Overweight?

Foundations come in three basic weights, or amounts of coverage: sheer, medium and full coverage. Most women look best in a sheer foundation, which lets most of the skin shine through, or a medium-weight makeup, which hides minor imperfections without appearing masklike. Don't routinely use a full-coverage foundation unless you need to hide a birthmark or other pigment problem. There are times when you may want to use a heavier foundation, however—in the winter, for example, for extra protection from wind and cold. Then switch to a lighter formulation in warmer weather.

Climate can determine the coverage you need, too. "Think of foundation as a fabric," says Manzoni. "If you live in Vancouver, where it's cold and dry, you'll need a heavier foundation than if you live in Miami, where it's hot and humid."

The Formula for Success

Are you oily-skinned and acne-prone? Or does your skin cry out for moisture? Whatever your skin type, here's how to choose the right foundation formula: oil-based, water-based or oil-free.

Oil-based foundations. Formulated with moisturizing ingredients like mineral oil, glycerin and lanolin, oil-based makeups—generally found in liquid or cream form—are best for dry or mature skin. "Oil-based foundations give mature skin a more supple, dewy look and won't call unnecessary attention to lines," says Geller.

Because oil-based makeups generally contain fewer skin-irritating preservatives and fragrances than other formulas, they usually suit sensitive skin, too. Almay and Clinique, among other companies, offer hypoallergenic, preservative- and fragrance-free foundations formulated for delicate complexions.

Water-based foundations. These lighter liquid or cream formulations usually list water as their first ingredient, but they still contain a small amount of oil or other emollient. The advantage to water-based foundations, however, is that they combine some moisturizing benefits in a matte (nonshiny) finish that's great for normal to slightly oily skin. You may want to choose an oil-free foundation, however, if your skin is extremely oily or blemish-prone.

The Scoop on Permanent Makeup

"Permanent makeup"—colored pigment tattooed on skin to simulate blusher, eyeliner or lipstick—is supposed to ensure that you can roll out of bed with bright cheeks, sparkling eyes and kissable lips. But while experts say a dermatologist or cosmetic surgeon experienced in the procedure can perform it safely, getting permanently made-up is not without risk—especially if you put your face in the wrong hands.

"There is a high risk of complications with permanent tattooing," says Paula A. Moynahan, M.D., attending plastic and reconstructive surgeon at Lenox Hill Hospital in New York City and St. Mary's Hospital and Waterbury Hospital in Waterbury, Connecticut. "The skin can become infected. Also, the tattoo could leach, meaning that the pigment doesn't stay where it's put—you could end up with a smudge rather than a fine line." Another potential risk of permanent makeup is allergic reactions to the pigments, especially those used by storefront operations.

If you are considering permanent makeup, it's *essential* that you choose a qualified dermatologist or cosmetic surgeon to perform the procedure. (Translation: Don't have it done by anyone else!) "Be sure he or she is experienced in performing permanent tattooing," says Dr. Moynahan. Check his or her credentials as well: A dermatologist should be certified by the American Academy of Dermatology and a cosmetic surgeon by the American Board of Plastic Surgery. Even so, considering all the risks, you're better off applying makeup the old-fashioned way. "I am emphatically against permanent tattooing. It's a no-go," says Albert M. Kligman, M.D., Ph.D.

Oil-free foundations. True to their name, oil-free makeups don't contain any emollients at all, which makes them a smart choice for oily or acne-prone skin. Some dermatologists scoff at the notion that the oil in some cosmetics aggravates acne, but if you tend to break out, why not use an oil-free foundation?

Cream-powder foundations. The newest and most versatile of the foundations, cream-powders are applied with a sponge or puff, with or without water: They go on light when used dry and heavier when applied wet. And virtually any skin type can use them: "They're especially good for oily skin that needs extra coverage," says Geller. And depending on which formula you choose, you may not need to use a separate concealer or powder.

The 60-Second Touch-Up

It's not your fault: Your makeup is bound to fade or sink into fine lines as you go through the day or evening. "We're talking about makeup on a living, breathing woman, not a latex finish on a wall," says New York makeup expert Pablo Manzoni. "That's why a quick touch-up in the ladies room is socially acceptable." Primp to perfection with these tips.

1. Blot shine with powder or a disposable filter paper.
2. Redistribute makeup that's settled into fine lines (under your eyes, for example) with a cotton swab or clean sponge.
3. Apply more cream blusher, if necessary. (If you use powder blusher, add it after step 4.)
4. Blot any remaining shine with translucent powder applied with a disposable cotton ball or pad.
5. Redistribute leftover lip pencil with a lip brush, then apply fresh lipstick from the tube or with your brush.

See also the chapter on lipsticks and other lip products (chapter 26) for lip pencil and lip-brush tips.

Be wary of these formulas if you have mature skin, however. Cream-powders that leave a matte finish can accentuate lines and wrinkles. Instead, look for products labeled *moisturizing* or *hydrating* that leave skin looking dewy.

When it comes to applying foundation, less really is more—and blending is everything. Follow this easy, step-by-step procedure.

1. Dip a cotton swab into your foundation bottle or stroke it along your compact. (It's more sanitary than using your fingers, says Geller.) Then place dime-size dots of foundation on your forehead, cheeks and chin.
2. Using your fingertips or a cosmetic sponge, blend foundation over your forehead, nose, cheeks and chin and under your eyes.
3. Blend well, especially at your jawline and around your ears.

A Pretty Flush of Blush

Blusher, usually found in cream, powder or cream-powder form, can brighten up your whole complexion. And you won't look clownish if you choose a blusher that compliments your skin tone and hair color, says Geller.

If you have fair skin and blonde hair, opt for soft, pale colors like coral or peach. Brunettes whose skin is more yellow than red look best in mocha, while ruddier brunettes should choose soft shades of coral. Pink, rosy or mauve blushers compliment gray hair, says Geller.

Black women with very dark, ashen skin can brighten their cheeks with hot-pink or fuchsia blusher, while shades of cinnamon, copper or rust flatter dark, mahogany-toned skin. Lighter-skinned black women should use orange-based shades.

But no matter which shade you choose, make sure your blusher's not too bright. An intense magenta or fuchsia cheek color may look pretty in the jar or compact, but the pigment in your skin can intensify a blusher's hue, imbuing your cheeks with two glaring spots instead of a subtle wash of color!

To avoid buying hues that are too vivid, try on a new blusher in daylight, even if you have to step outside the store. "Fluorescent lights may fool you into thinking a color is less intense than it is," says Geller. Also, try blushers on your bare skin, if possible; the worst time to shop for blusher is after work, when you have a day's worth of oil and old makeup on your face.

Cream or Powder?

As with foundation, choose a blusher formula with your skin type in mind.

Powder blushers suit oily complexions best because their matte finish won't contribute to shine. You might even investigate oil-free blushers.

The matte finish of a powder blusher is exactly what you don't need if you have drier or more mature skin, however. So choose a cream blusher: Its dewy finish will play down lines and wrinkles.

Cream-powder blushers combine the pliability of a cream with the brush-on ease of a powder and suit any skin type—even mature and oily complexions can wear them. "They're creamier than powder blushers but not at all greasy," says Geller.

How to Blush Beautifully

Remember that color belongs on the high point of your cheekbones. To find this point, smile broadly, then find the top of the swell with your fingers.

To apply cream blusher: Place a dime-size dot of blusher on each cheek with your fingertip or a cosmetic sponge and blend until you can't see where the blusher begins or ends. If you've applied too much color, gently wipe away the excess with a cosmetic sponge.

To apply powder or cream-powder blusher: Use a round brush just about the width of your cheeks. Touch the bristles of your brush to the cake and tap off excess color. Then apply lightly, blending with light, feathery strokes until you've softened any lines of demarcation. Dust translucent powder over your cheeks to tone down too-bright color.

Powder: The Final Touch

Face powder, which comes in loose and pressed forms, is generally just plain old talc and mineral oil. But it's indispensable to the perfectly done face: Loose power sets makeup and gives it a polished finish, while the heavier pressed powder soaks up oily shine or substitutes for foundation.

Some powders offer even more. "If you wear a sheer foundation or none at all, experiment with a loose tinted powder to even out your skin tone," says Geller. You might also use a frosted powder to give your skin an extra sparkle on special nights.

Pick-a-Powder

Today's face powder is as skin-specific as foundation. Decide what you want from your powder, then shop for the right product and the right applicator.

If You Want This	Try This
→ To set makeup	Loose transparent powder, applied with an oversize fluffy brush
→ To help control oil and shine	Oil-blotting powder, applied with a velour puff or sponge
→ To give dry skin a polished look	A moisturizing powder, applied with an oversize brush
→ To touch up makeup	Pressed powder (moisturizing formula for dry skin, oil-free/oil-blotting formula for oily skin), applied with disposable cotton pads
→ To help cover imperfections	A cream-powder formula (for dry, mature skin) or an oil-free extra-coverage formula (for oily skin), applied with a velour puff or sponge
→ To add a glow to mature skin	A lightly frosted or low-pearl powder, applied to the high point of the cheeks with an oversize fluffy brush

Know Your Skin Type

Powder? On dry skin? No way, you say. Actually, they're quite compatible—these days, there's a powder for every complexion.

If you have dry or mature skin, try a moisturizing product like Cover Girl's Replenishing Loose Powder. Apply with a brush for the lightest application, a dry sponge for more coverage and a wet sponge, in place of foundation, for maximum coverage.

But keep even wet powder away from lines or wrinkles, says Geller. "It tends to sink into fine lines, especially around your eyes, the sides of your mouth and above your upper lip," she says.

Oily complexions can opt for an oil-free powder or an oil-blotting powder like Coty Correctives, which delays shine by actually sensing and soaking up oil that reaches the surface of your skin. If you'd rather not load down oily skin with too many cosmetics, you can wear the Coty product instead of foundation.

You can also soak up oil with a quick pat of pressed powder. But to keep from looking chalky, limit your touch-ups to three or four a day. And to keep both your powder cake and your complexion fresh, apply your powder with disposable cotton pads. "If you keep using the same sponge, you'll transfer oils and bacteria to your face every time you use it," says Geller.

A quick, clean way to mop up midday accumulations of oil is to use oil-blotting papers, which you can tuck into your makeup bag. You can find these shine-stoppers dusted with a hint of powder; Geller suggests Papier Poudre, available at cosmetics stores or drugstores.

De-aging Makeup Hints

Used incorrectly, even the most expensive makeup will look less than flattering. So avoid these common—and easily correctable—cosmetic errors.

Lighten up! From foundation to powder, make up with a light hand (especially important as your skin matures). "Don't use too much makeup; it will look like you're trying to paint a new face," says Manzoni.

Do blend in. If your foundation stops at your jawline or your blusher just sits on top of your foundation, you have to blend! For flawless blending, use a clean sponge or a lamb's-wool paddle, available at beauty supply stores, says Geller. "Your fingers will just move your makeup around and around," she says.

See the light. Apply your makeup in natural light, if possible, using a magnifying mirror to make up and two mirrors to check your work from all angles. "Move those mirrors around to see what others will see," says Manzoni.

See also the chapter on sensitive skin (chapter 15).

CHAPTER TWENTY-SIX

Lipstick

Perfecting Your Pucker Power

The finishing touch to your makeup routine: a hasty dash of lipstick. Then you're out the door. Who has time to primp?

But hold on: Adding 60 seconds or so to your makeup routine can take your lip look from so-so to sensational. Even better, you don't have to spend $12, $15 or $20 on a lipstick to get beautiful results. Millions of women (including cover models) look great in $4 to $6 lipsticks they pick up at the drugstore.

It's cheap, it's fun, it brightens up your whole face . . . that's the beauty of lipstick. So find out how to make your lips their most alluring. All it takes is that one extra minute—and the right tools and techniques.

Lip Color: Made in the Shade

Faced with hundreds of shades of lipsticks to choose from, you may have no idea which hues are right for you. And months—or years—of trial and error can be expensive and frustrating.

Want to know the real secret to finding the right lipstick? Choose the right wardrobe. From there on in, it's a snap.

Your most flattering wardrobe colors will probably be your prettiest lipstick shades, says Laura Geller, makeup artist and owner of

Laura Geller Make-Up Studios, a cosmetics store in New York City. So if you know what your color is, you're halfway there. "No lip color is wrong if you like it and it blends with the clothing you're wearing," says Geller.

Generally speaking, if you wear a lot of pastels, you'll be safe with

What Are Your Prettiest Lip Colors?

To find the most flattering lip colors for your complexion, consult the table below.

Skin Tone	Choose	Never Use
Fair		
Blondes	Warm coral, peach and peachy-brown shades; orange-based reds	Bright reds, blue-red shades
Redheads	Peach, apricot, copper and bronze shades; other shades similar to hair color	Shades of pink
Olive	Rich pink, pink-red, soft corals	Peach and brown shades; blue-based reds
Ruddy	Soft coral and apricot shades	Pink-red and blue-red shades
Black		
Light skin	Deep wine, brown and burgundy shades	Orange shades
Darker skin	Brights: orange, red, pink, fuchsia shades; cream finish for sparkle and shine	Brown and wine shades; matte finish

soft lipstick colors. Favor bold colors like ruby red and sapphire blue? You'll probably look best in a red lipstick with a slight orange or blue undertone.

You'll also want to key your color choice to your skin tone (see "What Are Your Prettiest Lip Colors?"): Most likely, your skin is either more red (ruddy) or more yellow (sallow), and picking the shade that matches this undertone can warm up or cool down your complexion, says Geller.

"For example, if you have a lot of red in your skin, stay away from blue-based lipsticks, like fuchsia and ruby—these colors will make you look ruddier," says Geller. If your skin has more of a sallow undertone, avoid yellow-based hues like corals. When in doubt, go with a milder concentration of the color you like—a burnished rather than a scarlet red, for example.

If you have mature skin, wearing just a hint of lipstick can brighten up your whole face, says Geller. She suggests using clear, pure colors like pink or rose and avoiding muted shades like coral or burgundy. But avoid matte (nonshiny) finishes; they'll make your mouth look dry and your face tired. "You need a bit of gloss or the sheen of a cream lipstick to create a luminescence," says Geller.

Lip Color That Lasts and Lasts and Lasts . . .

"Why does the color fade so fast?" This beauty battle cry launched a thousand lipsticks (well, more than a few, at least) formulated to give lip color long-lasting cling.

The bad news: These long-lasting lipsticks often have matte finishes that dry out your lips or contain ingredients that stain lips, further drying them out.

Fortunately, more cosmetics companies are making more long-lasting lip colors with cream bases. The secret: micronizing, or pulverizing, the pigment (the ingredients that give lipstick its color and coverage) to almost invisible particles, which are then coated with moisturizers. The result: rich, creamy color that lasts. Revlon pioneered long-lasting, nondrying lip color with its Lipsexxxy lipsticks; Max Factor, Prescriptives and L'Oreal, among others, have followed suit.

If you can't find a long-lasting cream in a color you like, compromise with a semimatte lipstick, suggests Geller. "It's a bit longer-lasting than cream and moister than a straight matte," she says. "Or mix a matte lipstick with a little lipgloss, vitamin E stick or even petroleum jelly to make a matte formula more creamy."

But since nothing, not even your beloved Electric Pink lip color, lasts forever, be realistic about lipstick's staying power. "Women apply lipstick in the morning and expect it to last through lunch," says Sylvie Chantecaille, senior executive of creative marketing at Prescriptives in New York City. "It can last almost that long, but not quite."

If you use a lip pencil (see below) in the morning, however, a quick touch-up from the tube might be all you need to revive your lipstick after your plate of pasta.

Kiss Off Dry Lipstick

What good is the perfect shade of lipstick if it makes your lips look and feel like you've coated them with chalk? No good at all. That's why it pays to choose a moisture-rich lipstick formula.

You'll probably find that your lips get drier as you get older. So

Helping Lipstick Stay Put

Your first line of defense against bleeding (lipstick color seeping up into the fine lines above your upper lip) is using a lip pencil. If you still have problems or if your lipstick fades too quickly, prep your lips with a lip fixative or sealer, like Coty's Stop It! Anti-Feathering Stick for Lips and Max Factor's Stay Put Anti-Fade Lip Base.

"There are lots of different formulas in different strengths," explains Laura Geller, makeup artist and owner of Laura Geller Make-Up Studios, a cosmetics store in New York City. "Some are 'correctors' and look like stick concealers. The strongest ones are brush-on liquids."

For chronic bleeding, use a sealer daily. Or save it for busy days when you won't have time for touch-ups or for when you want your lip color to last the night.

give matte lipsticks the heave-ho and try cream formulations, which condition your lips. Cream formulas also soften the appearance of mature skin. "The softer your lips, the softer your whole appearance," says Geller.

You'll find creamy formulas by almost every major cosmetics company, including Avon, Max Factor and Revlon. You might also want to try L'Oreal's Colour Riche Hydrating Lipcolour, available in 48 shades.

You need to use a lip pencil before you apply cream lipsticks, however: Lipsticks can bleed, or seep up into the fine lines above your upper lip. "Creams can bleed and feather a lot quicker than matte lipsticks," says Geller, and a pencil will help keep color from going "outside the lines." (For more on beating the bleeding problem, see "Helping Lipstick Stay Put.")

Lip Tricks of the Trade

If you apply your lipstick straight from the tube, listen up: Precision counts.

A neat, finished look is more attractive and youthful-looking than an on-the-run application of color, says Chantecaille. "That means you should use a lip pencil and maybe even a lip brush," she says.

Makeup artists depend on these tools to give their clients' lips high-definition impact. You may have stopped using pencils and brushes because they add an extra step to your makeup routine or shied away from using them altogether, believing them too difficult to use. But with a little practice, lip pencils and brushes can help correct flaws and compensate for small but unwelcome changes that you may begin to notice as your lips mature.

"When you have a perfect lip-pencil application, your mouth is made," declares New York makeup expert Pablo Manzoni. Here's why: Lip pencils define the shape of your lips, help your lipstick last longer and prevent color from bleeding into feathery lines that often begin to appear above the lipline. What's more, using pencil in the morning gives you a touch-up guideline that lasts all day. As you'll see, a lip pencil even lets you redo the shape of your mouth.

As for the lip brush? Geller says it's one of her most important makeup tools. A lip brush lets you apply color more precisely than slicking on lipstick from the tube and helps set your first application of lip color of the day. "The lipstick you apply in the morning lasts the longest," says Geller. "It's the neatest and most definitive application of the day, so it pays to do it right."

You can also use a lip brush to touch up fading color when there's still some pencil definition left. Just apply the edge of the brush to your lipline and redistribute leftover pencil by blending it toward your mouth.

If you want to try a good lip brush without investing much cash, look for the Gold Leaf brand, available at beauty supply stores. The retractable styles work like ballpoint pens, so there's never a mess, even if the brush gets buried at the bottom of your bag. Revlon and Cover Girl also make easy-to-use lip brushes. And they last for years.

Sharpening Your Lip-Pencil Skills

Yes, you can pencil in the perfect mouth—it just takes practice. Just follow these simple lip tricks.

A fine line. Working from the center outward on your upper lip and from the corners inward on your lower lip, outline your lips with a thin pencil line. To make your lips fuller, line just the outside edge of lips and no more; to make them less full, line the area just within the lipline. You can steady your hand by resting your pinkie on your chin and your elbow on a steady surface like a countertop.

Next, go over your first thin line with a very thick application of pencil. Soften the color with a cotton swab, moving in toward your mouth. The swab removes excess pencil as it blends the line.

Load up on lip color. Apply your lipstick, preferably with a lip brush, right over the softened lip-pencil line. You shouldn't see the line at all when you're finished.

Pencil messes and misses. Don't use a lip pencil that's darker or—worse—a totally different shade than your lipstick (for example, brown pencil with pale pink lipstick). "Pencil color should harmonize with your lipstick shade," says Manzoni. Many cosmetics companies make lip pencils that match their lipsticks, so look for these foolproof partners.

CHAPTER TWENTY-SEVEN

Moisturizers

Smoother, Softer Skin at Any Age

Confused about the why, what, where, when and how of moisturizers? Join the club. Faced with such a dizzying array of high-tech and high-priced moisturizers—and so much hype—it can be pretty rough to choose a skin smoother!

So it may come as a relief to know that you don't have to spend a fortune on moisturizer. You just have to pick the formula that best suits your skin—and take the miracles with a grain of salt.

Tonics for Thirsty Skin

It doesn't matter whether you spend $40 or $4.99; virtually all moisturizers do what they're supposed to: soften your skin. "There's no such thing as a moisturizer that doesn't work," says Albert M. Kligman, M.D., Ph.D. "They all make your skin less dry."

Moisturizers protect your skin's top layer, the stratum corneum, by holding in water and smoothing surface dryness. They also prepare your skin for makeup, which glides on more easily and looks prettier on a smooth complexion. But most important, moisturizers make the skin on your face more supple, and supple skin hides its fine lines better.

Notice that it hides, not eliminates. Moisturizers absolutely do not prevent or get rid of wrinkles. That's why ads for moisturizers often claim that their products reduce the appearance of lines, not erase the lines themselves.

While moisturizers can't get rid of wrinkles, you can buy products formulated with ingredients thought to discourage them. Moisturizers formulated with alpha hydroxy acids (AHAs), mild acids derived from natural substances like fruit and milk, appear to make skin look smoother and brighter, while products that contain certain vitamins called antioxidants are thought—but not proven—to fight age-related skin damage caused by free radicals.

But the best wrinkle-deterring moisturizer ingredient money can buy is still a strong sunscreen, which guards your skin against photodamage.

Navigating the Moisturizer Maze

If you're over 25, you need a moisturizer. Or do you? "Probably the biggest misconception about moisturizers is that everyone needs one," says Stephen M. Purcell, D.O., chairman of the Division of Dermatology at the Philadelphia College of Osteopathic Medicine.

Whether you need a moisturizer depends on your skin type: oily, dry or a combination of both, says James N. Bollinger, Ph.D., associate director of pharmaceutical research and development at Galderma Laboratories in Fort Worth, Texas. In turn, "your skin type determines the type of moisturizer you need, from a thin lotion to a thick cream," he says.

Finding a moisturizer you love is a process of trial and error—and personal preference. Some women love to splurge on fancy moisturizers with all the trimmings; others prefer inexpensive, get-the-job-done products. Whichever you like, the best judge of whether a moisturizer works is you. "Your opinion counts," says Mitchell S. Wortzman, Ph.D., president of Neutrogena Dermatologics in Los Angeles. "Your moisturizer should satisfy these two questions: Do I think it works? and Does my skin feel better?"

Moisturizing oily skin. Good news for the shiny-faced: You may not have to use a moisturizer at all, because your skin's natural oils may protect it from water loss. In fact, using a moisturizer when you don't need one could actually create a problem, like blemishes. "Yogi Berra's famous quip, 'If it ain't broke, don't fix it,' applies here," says Dr. Purcell.

That doesn't mean oily skin can't feel dry—often the result of over-cleansing (a knee-jerk response to oiliness) or stripping your skin with alcohol-based products like astringents. Try cleansing your skin more gently and see if the dryness goes away.

If your skin still feels parched, a moisturizer that contains humectants (ingredients that attract and hold water) like glycerin, sodium PCA and hyaluronic acid can help. An oil-free, humectant-type moisturizer like Nivea's No Oil, All Moisture Hydrogel will trap water and soften your skin's top layer without adding oiliness or shine.

Quenching normal to dry skin. Pick a moisturizer formulated with emollients like triglycerides, oils, petrolatum and silicone, recommends Dr. Bollinger.

The drier your skin, the more oil your moisturizer should contain.

A Little Dab Will Dew Ya

If you're reluctant to spend your hard-earned dollars on high-priced moisturizers, head to your medicine cabinet: The ultimate emollient, or skin softener, is plain old petroleum jelly. Many dermatologists give it high marks as a moisturizer, although it's admittedly on the order of greasy kid stuff if you use too much.

Try smoothing on a dab of petroleum jelly as a before-bed treatment, especially during the winter, to ease the drying effects of most heating systems. To get the benefits of petroleum jelly without sliding off your pillow, simply wipe it off after a minute or two, says Lorraine H. Kligman, Ph.D., associate research professor in the Department of Dermatology at the University of Pennsylvania School of Medicine in Philadelphia. "There will still be enough left on your skin to do you some good overnight," she says.

An added bonus: Not only is petroleum jelly dirt cheap, it's a godsend to people with supersensitive skin who sometimes react to even the most innocuous ingredients in many moisturizers.

If your skin's only slightly to moderately dry, choose a moisturizer that contains more water than oil or an oil-in-water emulsion, says Dr. Wortzman. To find one, check the product's label and consistency: Water will lead the list of ingredients, and the moisturizer will be very fluid.

If your skin is very dry, you'll need a moisturizer formulated with more oil than water, or a water-in-oil emulsion. An oil compound is generally first on the list of ingredients, and the moisturizer's consistency is very thick, "almost like petroleum jelly," says Dr. Wortzman.

Keep in mind that the more oil a moisturizer contains, the longer it takes to dry.

Day Creams/Night Creams/Eye Creams: Who Needs What

If you have as many face creams as lipsticks, you'll be glad to know you can streamline that collection of bottles and jars. "For the most part, one moisturizer should be sufficient for most skin types," says Dr. Purcell.

Some cosmetics companies agree with that assessment and have introduced around-the-clock moisturizers that preclude the need for a separate day, night or eye cream. In other words, you don't have to buy one product for your face, another for your neck and yet another for under your eyes: Products like Prescriptives All You Need Action Moisturizer and Clinique Turnaround Cream are meant to go under your makeup by day and to be used alone at night.

But be sure you read the labels to know what you're getting in an all-in-one moisturizer—or not getting. Case in point: All You Need has the exfoliating benefits of AHAs, but no sunscreen.

So springing for a separate day, night or eye cream may appeal to you. Here's how each product adds up.

Daytime moisturizers. These light creams or lotions generally soak into your skin in about five minutes, so you can apply your makeup without waiting around for your face to dry.

The best reason to use a daytime moisturizer is to give your skin the benefit of a product with added sunscreen—the higher the sun protection factor (SPF), the better, so consider a moisturizer with an SPF of at least 15. You'll find many products that fit the bill; two to consider are Eucerin Daily Facial Lotion SPF 20 or Pond's Nourishing Moisturizer with SPF 15.

Smooth on a daytime moisturizer while your skin is still damp from cleansing so the product can trap moisture. Apply your make-up when the moisturizer no longer feels sticky on your face.

Night creams. Oilier and thicker than daytime moisturizers, night creams are usually too greasy to go under makeup by day—which is why they're perfect for use at bedtime. Inexpensive standards like Nivea Creme and petroleum jelly fit the bill, but you can also try Neutrogena Light Night Cream, L'Oreal Plenitude Advanced Overnight Replenisher and Pond's Overnight Moisturizing Complex.

Eye creams. Do you really need an eye-specific cream? It depends on whom you ask. Some dermatologists feel they're a waste of money and that using your regular moisturizer under your eyes is just fine. Other dermatologists suggest using a bona fide eye cream if you have sensitive skin or your eyes are easily irritated. But be aware: These eye-specific moisturizers contain certain preservatives that could be irritating.

Taking the Acid Test

So far, no one's managed to bottle the fountain of youth. But cheer up: The cosmetic chemists keep trying. If you're willing to settle for slightly less than a miracle, though, you might try a moisturizer formulated with AHAs. Derived from natural substances like fruit (citric acid), sugar cane (glycolic acid) and milk (lactic acid), these mild acids are making their way into more and more moisturizers and have received much beauty industry and word-of-mouth buzz.

Not entirely without cause: AHAs appear to smooth and brighten skin by increasing cell turnover and by sloughing off dead cells that dull the skin's top layer.

AHAs also chemically change the structure of the skin's outer layer so it holds water better, says Dr. Purcell. "As a result, the skin looks and feels more supple," he says. Some dermatologists even believe AHAs can eliminate fine lines and wrinkles.

Most over-the-counter moisturizers contain very low percentages of AHAs—generally 4 to 8 percent. A dermatologist can prescribe moisturizers with slightly higher concentrations of the acids. Lac-Hydrin 12, for example, contains 12 percent lactic acid.

But here's the big question: Does more AHA equal more benefit? While some dermatologists say even the small amounts of AHAs in over-the-counter moisturizers may improve the appearance of your skin, dermatologists haven't yet determined whether the more-is-better theory is valid, according to Dr. Purcell.

"Nobody really knows what percentage of an AHA in a product works best," says Dr. Purcell. "We recommend a 12 percent product because we figure you're getting the maximum benefit. But it's never been proven that a 12 percent concentration works better than a 10 percent or even a 4 percent product."

One thing's for sure: AHA-enhanced moisturizers have been wildly popular, and many women love them, fulfilling both of Dr. Wortz-man's criteria for testing a moisturizer's effectiveness. But in the final analysis, you'll have to take the acid test for yourself.

Also, you should know that two or three years after AHAs were first introduced, questions about their long-term safety arose. Frequent use, it seems, may exhaust the skin's natural ability to repair itself. Until the risks are confirmed (or disproved), check with your dermatologist before using AHAs.

Can Antioxidants Help You Save Face?

Will rubbing certain vitamins into your skin really slow your skin's aging process and help repair sun damage? Probably not. But that hasn't stopped cosmetics companies from adding vitamins A, C and E, also known as antioxidants, to their moisturizers.

Antioxidants search for and destroy free radicals—so-called bad cells generated by natural body functioning and by smoke, pollution and sunlight. "Free radicals certainly damage cells and contribute to aging," says Dr. Kligman.

What causes free-radical damage in the first place? In a word, oxidation. The same chemical process that causes fruit to turn soft and spotty and metal to rust, oxidation also breaks down the skin's elastin and collagen, the stuff that keeps it youthfully firm.

The logic behind adding antioxidants to moisturizers sounds reasonable: If ingesting them prevents age-related damage internally, then slathering them directly on the skin will work even better. Yet there's little evidence to suggest that rubbing antioxidants into your skin really helps.

"Antioxidants ought to work, but it hasn't been demonstrated beyond a doubt," says Dr. Kligman. "Skin-care products that contain antioxidants still need more testing to prove that they really work."

Some vitamin-based creams do have skin-rejuvenating properties, like Retin-A (topical tretinoin), the vitamin A–derived cream used to treat acne and fight wrinkles, and a vitamin C cream (still in the test stage) that seems to guard skin against sun damage. But these creams are formulated differently than over-the-counter products, have undergone rigorous testing and are classified as drugs, not cosmetics.

Special Delivery for Your Skin

The way some moisturizers deliver their ingredients supposedly helps them penetrate more deeply into your skin, but again, there's no scientific evidence to prove it.

Some moisturizer formulas capture their ingredients in little globules called liposomes, designed to somehow burst at just the right time and in just the right way on your skin. Other delivery systems you see advertised—like nanospheres, encapsulation or microsponges—work along the same principle.

But Dr. Kligman believes liposomes are too large for your skin to absorb: "If you can get a liposome through the top layer of your skin, you can get an elephant through a doorway," he claims.

So whether a moisturizer releases its ingredients in bubbles or bursts shouldn't sway you when you're at the cosmetics counter, according to Dr. Kligman. "First, it's not certain if liposomes make ingredients significantly more effective," he says. "Second, many companies have already jumped on the bandwagon. High-tech formulas will soon be commonplace rather than a source of distinction."

See also the chapters on cleansers (chapter 22) and wrinkle creams (chapter 29).

CHAPTER TWENTY-EIGHT

Sunscreen

The All-Season Accessory

Although you usually won't find it packaged in a fancy bottle and displayed prominently on drugstore shelves, sunscreen is the best antiwrinkle cosmetic you can buy. Why? Because sun damage is the leading cause of wrinkled, rough, blotchy skin. In fact, many experts say that age spots, wrinkles and other signs associated with not-so-young skin are the direct cumulative result of decades of unprotected sun exposure, rather than of aging itself.

The problem is ultraviolet (UV) rays—a form of radiation, really—that penetrate the skin, invading the normally sturdy layers below and eventually destroying collagen and elastin. Collagen makes your skin firm and youthfully plump. Elastin gives skin resiliency and keeps expression lines from forming into creases and wrinkles.

But there's more than, well, a ray of hope for your complexion. No matter what your age, you can help prevent further sun damage by using a strong sunscreen—lotions, gels, creams and oils formulated to absorb sunlight so your skin doesn't. You might even opt for a sunblock, which protects your skin even more. On the other hand, it's important to understand what sunscreens and sunblocks can't do.

The Deciding Factor

A sunscreen's SPF, or sun protection factor, represents a multiple of how long you can stay in the sun without burning. If you burn within 15 minutes of being exposed to the sun with no protection, for example, wearing a sunscreen with SPF 15 would theoretically allow you to stay in the sun for 225 minutes (3¾ hours) before you started to burn.

But sunscreens don't make sunning safe, because sunscreen alone won't keep the sun from aging your skin. "You can still get sun damage even if you use a good sunscreen," says Albert M. Kligman, M.D., Ph.D. "Some rays will get through."

The trouble is, the sun penetrates your skin through even the strongest sunscreens. "It's simply a matter of time," explains Dr. Kligman. "You can spend a week in Miami, use an SPF 15 product and not show much of a tan. But stay there three or four weeks and you'll tan quite a bit."

In other words, while sunscreens can help keep you from burning, they only delay tanning—a slower form of sun damage. What's more, sun damage is cumulative: Lines, rough skin texture and blotches won't show up on your face for years.

Fortunately, the word is out that tanned skin is sun-damaged skin. "You'll get fewer wrinkles and blotches if you use a sunscreen," says Dr. Kligman. That's why sun-protection products fly off the shelves, moisturizers with added sunscreen sell like hotcakes and women of all ages are sporting pale faces in August.

And don't fall prey to the fallacy that dark skin is more immune to sun damage, either. Even African Americans, whose skin contains more melanin (the substance that gives skin its pigment and also causes it to tan), can get sun damage. For that matter, so can people of Mediterranean ancestry and others with moderate degrees of pigmentation.

But don't press your luck, warns Dr. Kligman. "Many people, especially those of Northern European ancestry, shouldn't depend entirely on sunscreens if they're working outdoors or otherwise spending a lot of time in the sun," he says.

While no sunscreen can offer you complete protection, there is reason to believe that slathering on a strong sunscreen regularly may help prevent skin cancer. An Australian study by the Anti-Cancer Council of Victoria tracked 431 patients with precancerous growths who were assigned, at random, to use an SPF 17 sunscreen. After seven months, patients who'd used the sunscreen saw 24 percent of their growths shrink or disappear, while the people who didn't saw slightly less improvement.

More good news: Using sunscreen doesn't seem to lead to a deficiency in vitamin D, which your body produces when it's exposed to sunlight. The same Australian study found that, after seven months, people who used sunscreen had as much vitamin D in their blood as those who didn't.

Screening Out Wrinkles

You're baking in the sun and feeling virtuous: You're slathered with a sunscreen whose label sports a double-digit SPF number.

Good for you, right? Right—except that your sunscreen may be

Sunning by the Numbers

A good rule of thumb: Wear sunscreen every day, rain or shine. The question is, how strong a product do you need?

SPF 15: Everyday protection. Many dermatologists recommend using a sun protection factor (SPF) of 15 all the time, whatever the climate or season. So get your daily dose of SPF 15 in a regular sunscreen or moisturizers or foundations with added sunscreens.

SPF 30: Extra protection. If you're planning an all-day jaunt to the beach, park or golf course, use a sunblock or sunscreen with an SPF of up to 30. Use these industrial-strength sunscreens as a matter of course if you have very fair skin and burn or freckle easily or are located closer to the equator or at higher altitudes, where the sun's rays are most intense.

Yet there's no need to go overboard with an SPF of 40 or 50: Most dermatologists feel that SPFs over 30 don't provide much additional protection.

filtering out only a fraction of the sun's damaging rays.

You're exposed to two kinds of ultraviolet light: ultraviolet-B (UVB), the so-called burning rays, which are more prevalent in summer and strongest at midday, and ultraviolet-A (UVA), which aren't as strong as UVB but reach the earth year-round and in greater amounts. At one time, experts thought only UVB caused skin cancer and photoaging. It now appears that UVA can lead to both of these skin villains, just more slowly than UVB.

UVA also passes through clouds and glass—and most sunscreens, many of which absorb only UVB. (More about why later.) The upshot: It's vital to protect your health as well as your complexion with a strong sunscreen that absorbs both UVB and UVA.

Sunscreens: What Works—And Why

So you're convinced you don't want to play the frying game. But to choose the sun protection product that's best for you, you need to know just what's out there. So here's a rundown of your sun-shield options and how they work.

Classic sunscreens. The basic sunscreen, in cream, lotion or oil form, contains chemicals that absorb sunlight. PABA (short for para-aminobenzoic acid), once the most common chemical sunscreen, fell out of favor as increasing numbers of people using it experienced skin irritation and rashes. Although PABA's still being used (it's a good chemical sunscreen), most sunscreens now contain padimate-O, cinnamates and salicylates, which are less likely to irritate your skin.

Unfortunately, most chemical sunscreens still absorb only UVB light, allowing UVA to penetrate your skin. In fact, that SPF number on your bottle of sunscreen refers only to its UVB protection.

But that's changing. Now that dermatologists consider UVA a threat, a few sunscreens have added ingredients like oxybenzone or other benzophenones—which absorb some UVA—to their UVB-screening formulas. So far, the only chemical sunscreen that provides substantial protection against both UVA and UVB is Shade UVAGUARD, formulated with the best UVA zapper to date—Parsol 1789, or avobenzone.

What may not work: synthetic melanin. Some cosmetics companies have added it to their sunscreens to simulate the protection offered by the melanin naturally present in heavily pigmented skin. This artificial pigment appears to have limited, if any, value, however, since melanin is only a stopgap measure to protect skin from burning: Synthetic melanin can't prevent sun damage. In any case, there's no scientific evidence that smearing on melanin works. "Many of these products contain chemical sunscreens," notes Dr. Kligman, which may be providing the real sun protection.

Physical-barrier sunscreens. Remember how your grandmother used to bundle up at the beach—hat, sunglasses, umbrella, the works? You might think of these products as your own invisible sun umbrella. Physical-barrier sunscreens act as shields, screening out both UVB and UVA. And because physical-barrier products work immediately, you can step into the sun right after you slather them on.

When Is a Sunblock Not a Sunblock?

Some sunscreen manufacturers have played fast and loose with the terms *sunscreen* and *sunblock*. But the Food and Drug Administration (FDA) is gearing up to change the way these sun products are labeled.

Strictly speaking, a sunblock uses a physical barrier like zinc oxide or titanium dioxide to screen all ultraviolet light. Sunscreens absorb only some rays—mostly ultraviolet-B— while letting others penetrate your skin.

Although the difference between the two products seems apparent, regulations by the FDA allow sunscreens with SPF numbers of 12 or above to be labeled sunblocks. One of many FDA proposals under consideration is that a sun product must contain a physical barrier to have the word *sunblock* on its label.

The FDA's final rulings on the safe use of sunscreen and product labeling are several years away. Until then, read the back of your sunscreen (block?) bottle to see whether or not your "sunblock" contains titanium dioxide or zinc oxide.

The most effective physical-barrier ingredient is zinc oxide, the gunky white paste made famous by generations of lifeguards. Its appearance is no longer a drawback, however. Zinc oxide can now be micronized, or reduced to virtually invisible particles. Of course, if you're the flamboyant type, you can wear brightly colored zinc oxide, available in drugstores, in shades like hot pink and yellow.

Another physical barrier, titanium dioxide, doesn't screen out as much UVA as its more powerful cousin zinc oxide. Many sun protection products combine titanium dioxide, which is also micronized, with zinc oxide to provide more protection than titanium dioxide alone.

Zinc oxide and titanium dioxide are also found in products containing chemical sunscreens. But now you can find completely chemical-free physical-barrier formulas more to your liking, especially if you have sensitive skin: They don't sting and burn the way chemical formulas can. For true chemical-free sunning, try Neutrogena Chemical-Free Sunblocker SPF 17 or Johnson & Johnson's Sundown Sport Sunblock. (Estee Lauder, Revlon and Chanel also make chemical-free blocks.) And one product—Eutra Block—is advertised as being chemical-, fragrance- and alcohol-free.

Whichever sun protection you choose, however, read a sunscreen's label carefully to make sure you know whether you're buying sun*screen* or sun*block*. While one company may offer a dozen different sun products, the packaging can look the same.

Screening Smart

How well a sunscreen protects your skin depends on how well you use it. Here's how to get the most from your sun protection.

Stay away from midday sun. Avoid the sun between 10:00 A.M. and 3:00 P.M., when the sun's rays are strongest.

Slather on sunscreen early. Apply a sunscreen a half-hour before you go out to allow it to penetrate your skin's top layer, and 15 minutes before you apply makeup.

Sunblock protection starts as soon as you apply it, but it's still a good idea to rub it in before you go out. Read the label for reapplication instructions.

Don't be stingy. To get a sunscreen's full protection, you have to use the right amount. Experts recommend using about an ounce of lotion per application to cover your entire body. So don't expect that four-ounce bottle to last the whole summer.

But even if you're only buying enough sunscreen for a three-day jaunt, check the expiration date; sunscreen has a limited shelf life. That advice goes double for lotions that have been sitting in your bathroom closet or beach bag since your last sunny vacation.

Take sunscreen to the extreme. Smooth on sunscreen everywhere your bare flesh is exposed—every day. "I'm amazed at how many legs I see with sun damage," says Dr. Kligman. "Any place that's exposed is at risk." And who wants baggy knees when you get older? Protect the backs of your hands and your forearms, too.

Apply sunscreen under your clothes, too, if you'll be outdoors all day. The sun can penetrate some fabrics, especially bathing suits and cotton shirts, burning your less exposed, most vulnerable skin.

Keep the sunscreen flowing. Sunscreens fade away when you swim, towel off after a swim and perspire—even while you're just basking by the pool. "An SPF 15 might be only SPF 8 an hour later," says Dr. Kligman. So keep covering up with sunscreen.

Reapply after you take the plunge. Water-resistant is not waterproof, and even waterproof formulas expire. Most water-resistant formulas need to be reapplied after 80 minutes in the water. Sunblocks are more water-resistant, but recoat yourself anyway after a long dip or if you're sweating heavily.

Don't forget your lips. Unprotected lips can get badly burned, and repeated exposure to the sun can leave lips less than alluring. So carry a tube of SPF 15 lip sunscreen in your bag—and use it often.

Hide your eyes. Give your eyes their own sunscreen—sunglasses that block as much ultraviolet light as possible. The American National Standards Institute has set label standards: "Special purpose" lenses must block at least 99 percent of UVB light and "general purpose" lenses 95 percent. Prescription lenses can be treated to block UV light. It's a fact that wearing the proper eye protection helps prevent you from developing cataracts, as well as unattractive squint lines.

Go under cover. Stay in shady areas, wear a wide-brimmed hat to protect your scalp and further shield your eyes and sit under an umbrella if you can. "But don't think that hiding from the sun can replace using a sunscreen," warns Dr. Kligman.

Shun alcohol-based sunscreens. You're better off avoiding these formulas altogether; they don't seem to work as well and tend to sting your eyes more than other sunscreens. Worse, they're flammable, and they say so right on the label. So don't use them if you'll be barbecuing or sitting around a campfire.

Be mindful of your medication. Some prescription drugs can make you exquisitely sensitive to sunlight, leaving you with what looks and feels like a bad sunburn if you go out unprotected while taking the medication. Antibiotics are one example. "Fortunately, these reactions are rare," says Dr. Kligman. "But if you're taking any prescription drug, ask your doctor or pharmacist if you also need to take special precautions against the sun."

CHAPTER TWENTY-NINE

Wrinkle Creams

Don't Fall for a Line

*I*n a muddle over moisturizers? Then you're probably equally confused by so-called wrinkle creams. Ads for both of these products talk a lot about wrinkle reduction, so it's getting harder to tell the two apart.

It's even harder not to be tempted by the promises in wrinkle-cream ads, especially the ones that claim various degrees of wrinkle improvement by percentage. The unhappy fact is, nothing you can buy at the beauty counter will eliminate wrinkles.

But don't fret—there are ways to sort through the various options and find a product you're happy with. The key to satisfaction is a little lesson in chemistry combined with realistic expectations.

A War of Words

Much like moisturizers, most wrinkle creams work to improve the appearance of lines and wrinkles—to make them less noticeable, not make them disappear.

The fact is, wrinkles appear when the deeper layers of your skin have been damaged by a variety of factors, including the sun (especially the sun), smoking and gravity.

"Serious wrinkles form beneath the top layer of your skin," says Albert M. Kligman, M.D., Ph.D. "Wrinkles are caused by damage to your skin's collagen and elastin, supportive fibers in the dermis. That's why wrinkle creams can't really tackle the problem—they can deliver only surface help."

But that doesn't stop cosmetics companies from suggesting that their wrinkle creams can help rejuvenate your skin. While the government's cracked down on misleading and even downright fraudulent advertising in recent years, you still have to read between the lines to figure out what these wrinkle-cream ads are actually saying—and whether their suggestions are altogether truthful.

To avoid being targeted by the Food and Drug Administration (FDA), some companies have reined in their extravagant claims and promises. But ironically enough, other companies purposely understate their product's effect on wrinkles. Here's why: Any product that claims it can change the structure of your skin (for instance, by eliminating wrinkles) must be categorized as a drug, and drugs are subject to FDA review—an expensive, time-consuming proposition that cosmetics companies don't want to get into. Translation? You can't tell which over-the-counter wrinkle cream might work better than another.

The Acid Test

The newest wrinkle creams are actually moisturizers formulated with the beauty ingredient of the 1990s, alpha hydroxy acids (AHAs), mild acids derived from fruit, milk, sugar cane or other natural compounds. The two most common AHAs in moisturizers and wrinkle creams are glycolic acid, derived from sugar cane, and lactic acid, from milk. While most dermatologists agree that AHAs act as exfoliants (which slough off dead skin cells) and help skin trap moisture, some experts believe that these acids have some de-wrinkling powers, too.

And just how might these miracle ingredients succeed where so many contenders have failed? Eugene J. Van Scott, M.D., clinical professor of dermatology at Hahnemann University School of Medicine in Philadelphia, who's considered the father of AHAs, thinks these acids have the potential to plump up the dermis and substantially improve fine lines, and they may even improve the appearance of deeper wrinkles.

But it's important to note that Dr. Van Scott's patients were treated with strong concentrations of glycolic acid—in-office peels contained up to 70 percent and at-home prescriptions from 5 to 15 percent. By contrast, most over-the-counter products contain only 4 to 12 percent glycolic acid. So it's hard to say whether a consumer, using a weaker formula, would get the same kind of results Dr. Van Scott saw in his patients.

Says Jeffrey H. Binstock, M.D., assistant clinical professor of dermatologic surgery at the University of California at San Francisco, "As moisturizers, AHAs are quite nice. But whether they can actually help your skin to have fewer lines and wrinkles is another story."

Other dermatologists, however, feel that the cumulative effect of even a low concentration of AHAs might improve fine wrinkles. James J. Leyden, M.D., professor of dermatology at the University of Pennsylvania School of Medicine in Philadelphia, has studied Avon's Anew, which contains 4 percent glycolic acid (you can now buy it in an 8 percent formulation, too) and reports that those who've tried it say it helps. And according to Stephen M. Purcell, D.O., chairman of the Division of Dermatology at the Philadelphia College of Osteopathic Medicine, "The 4 percent in Anew will work better than the same cream without the glycolic acid." Both low-concentration creams usually take from four to six weeks to produce visible improvement, if any.

Lose Your Lines the Old-Fashioned Way

If the high price of wrinkle creams is putting a furrow in your brow, try a product straight from your grandmother's vanity table: Nivea cream, which contains mineral oil, petrolatum, glycerin and lanolin—all heavy-duty emollients.

"It's an old-fashioned product," says Albert M. Kligman, M.D., Ph.D. "There's nothing special in it, but, in my opinion, it does help reduce fine wrinkles moderately."

How or why Nivea can help reduce fine lines remains a mystery, says Dr. Kligman. "No one's done any 20-year studies, where one group puts it on and the other group doesn't," he says. But if you prefer to take a more modern approach to fighting wrinkles, the prescription product Retin-A is still your best bet.

How much improvement can you expect? It's impossible to predict, considering the continued debate about whether AHAs affect wrinkles at all. But many women have given moisturizers formulated with AHAs rave reviews. So while fine lines might stay put, using an AHA might improve the appearance of your skin itself.

If you want to try a cream formulated with an AHA, you can try an inexpensive, nonprescription cream like Lacticare, Lac-Hydrin 5, Aqua Glycolic Lotion or Eucerin Plus Creme. A dermatologist can prescribe products that contain higher concentrations of the acids. Either way, you should be aware that using a product containing an AHA may sting until your skin gets used to its strong exfoliating action.

A Is for Action

Critics of AHAs point to a lack of well-controlled clinical studies that prove AHAs work. First-hand reports of success, while potentially persuasive, are not considered scientific. So far, the only product with a scientifically proven track record is Retin-A (topical tretinoin), the vitamin A–derived prescription formula created by Dr. Kligman. At this writing, it's the best wrinkle treatment you can get in a tube, but it's only available by prescription. The active ingredient is tretinoin, a form of vitamin A.

Originally developed as an acne drug (it unplugs the clogged pores of problem skin), Retin-A's skin-renewal properties came as a surprise and still can't be explained. "Retin-A is a molecule that has the remarkable ability to stimulate all the cells in the dermis. They're all somehow 'turned on,' including the cells that make collagen," says Dr. Kligman.

Retin-A also gets rid of wrinkles without damaging the skin, adds Lorraine H. Kligman, Ph.D., associate research professor in the Department of Dermatology at the University of Pennsylvania School of Medicine in Philadelphia. Best of all, Retin-A's results remained even after women stopped using it for ten weeks.

Dr. Albert Kligman is realistic about Retin-A's limitations, however. "It works best on fine wrinkles," he says. "When you get the deep valleys, surgery is the only treatment that works."

Retin-A also makes the skin more vulnerable to sunlight. So if you choose Retin-A, you'll have to use sunscreen and avoid the sun, otherwise you'll get the worst sunburn of your life and damage your rejuvenating skin. Even without sun exposure, this drug can also cause redness and flaking of the skin. Using a moisturizer usually eases these side effects.

In fact, many dermatologists use Retin-A and an AHA in tandem: Retin-A at night and the AHA product in the morning. The AHA counteracts some of the Retin-A's irritation and helps the Retin-A to perform better: Melvin L. Elson, M.D., medical director of the Dermatology Center in Nashville and co-author of *The Good Look Book*, describes their combined action as "one plus one equals three."

The next generation of Retin-A, Renova, has a moisturizer already in it. Renova is awaiting FDA approval.

Ingredients: The Name Game

Some wrinkle creams contain ingredients that sound like they work. Collagen injections temporarily plump wrinkles, but collagen in a cream doesn't. Retin-A can improve wrinkles, but vitamin A in over-the-counter creams probably can't. And while retinol, the alcohol form of vitamin A, is added to many cosmetics, most products don't contain enough of it to give you Retin-A's results, explains Dr. Lorraine Kligman.

The same is true for retinyl compounds like retinyl palmitate and retinyl acetate, other vitamin A ingredients. To be effective, the concentrations of these ingredients would have to be higher.

More troubling than ingredients that do nothing are those that can actually harm your skin. Stay away from wrinkle creams that say they temporarily plump up wrinkles. Many do so by causing a low-grade inflammation and edema (swelling) that puffs up the creases—hardly a safe way to smooth out your skin.

"You see the softening and blurring of the wrinkles—it looks like they're going down. But what you don't see is the damage caused by using this kind of product for years," warns Dr. Albert Kligman.

See also the chapter on Retin-A (chapter 51).

PART THREE

Nutritional Maintenance for Beautiful Skin

CHAPTER THIRTY

Water and Healthy Skin

The Great H₂O Debate

"For beautiful skin, drink eight glasses of water a day." If you're like many women, you've heard this unproven—but enduring—bit of beauty lore time and time again. But can drinking 64 ounces of water a day—two quarts—really give skin a fresh, radiant glow?

The answer is . . . maybe. While most nutritional experts recommend sipping at least eight eight-ounce glasses of water every day, most dermatologists say there's no magic number that specifically benefits the skin. On the other hand, many women—including top models—claim that drinking lots of water helps prevent or clear blemishes and promotes a smooth, glowing complexion.

If you currently sip more soft drinks or coffee than plain water, there's no doubt that following the eight-a-day formula can benefit your health. And should you find that one of the rewards of drinking more water is a more radiant complexion, so much the better. But if you want the facts before you fill up, read on. Here's what the experts say about the water/skin connection.

How Much Is Enough?

You can only last about a week without water. This life-sustaining nutrient helps the body digest food, eliminate waste, regulate its temperature and lubricate its joints, among other functions. "A 120-pound woman has about 36 quarts of fluid in her body," says Susan M. Kleiner, R.D., Ph.D., a Seattle-based nutritionist and author of *The High Performance Cookbook*. "In a moderate climate, she can lose 2½ quarts per day just through perspiration and excretion. So for the average woman, drinking eight to ten cups of water a day merely replaces the water she's lost."

The skin needs water to maintain the body's moist internal environment. "The skin reflects our general health, and the body has to get enough water," says Melvin L. Elson, M.D., medical director of the Dermatology Center in Nashville and co-author of *The Good Look Book*.

But can filling up on water make skin glow? Some dermatologists think so. "Drinking lots and lots of water is wonderful for the skin," says Marianne O'Donoghue, M.D., associate professor of dermatology at Rush Presbyterian–St. Luke's Medical Center in Chicago. "Water keeps the body 'flushed.' "

Designer Water: A Matter of Taste

Many people associate bottled water with the bubbling mountain stream or icy glacier on its label. But unless your home water supply is contaminated for some reason, fancy bottled water isn't any purer than plain old tap water, says Susan M. Kleiner, R.D., Ph.D., a Seattle-based nutritionist and author of *The High Performance Cookbook*.

But you may find so-called designer water easier to swallow. Most people drink bottled water—a catch-all term for various products, including spring water, distilled water, sparkling water and mineral water—because they like the way it tastes (or doesn't taste). The chief difference among bottled waters is their mineral content: Some brands have more minerals, some have less, and some, like distilled and purified water, have none.

Some bottled waters also contain a high amount of sodium. So if you need to monitor your sodium intake for medical reasons, check labels.

But most dermatologists doubt that sipping a set amount of water can have a positive effect on your complexion. "I've never seen convincing evidence that drinking a certain number of glasses of water will benefit the skin," says Barbara Gilchrest, M.D., professor and chairman of dermatology at Boston University Medical Center. Says Albert M. Kligman, M.D., Ph.D., "There's no magic number—four glasses of water a day is usually enough."

Nor can water remedy specific skin conditions, say experts. "If you're a normal, healthy person and your skin's starting to look slightly wrinkled and dry, it's unlikely that you're going to correct the dryness by drinking water," says Dr. Gilchrest. "If you could, the cosmetics industry would be out of business." As for blemishes, "drinking water doesn't have a beneficial effect on acne," says Dr. Elson.

But as mentioned, many women claim that drinking more water means fewer blemishes. One woman, for example, finds that her skin begins to break out if she's neglected to drink enough water. So for three or four days, she drinks eight eight-ounce glasses of water a day. In two or three days, her complexion has begun to clear.

Easy Ways to Wet Your Whistle

Most nutritionists, including Dr. Kleiner, recommend that you drink water straight rather than get it through other fluids like soft drinks, juice or soup. Coffee and tea don't count either, says Dr. Kleiner. They contain caffeine, a common diuretic, which rids the body of water.

If the thought of drinking two quarts of water every day makes you queasy, relax. Meeting the quota isn't hard if you space your water intake over the course of the day. These tips from Dr. Kleiner can help make it easier to fill up without floating away.

Gulp water from bigger glasses. Using a 12- or 16-ounce tumbler means you only have to drink four or six glasses each day. This psychological trick works for some people; it might work for you.

Take water on the road ... Buy a cyclist's water bottle and keep it in your bag or car. It's fashionable and practical.

... and keep it handy. To remind yourself to drink up, set a big water bottle or pitcher on your desk during the day, on your coffee table in the evening and on your nightstand when you go to bed.

Stop and sip. Every time you pass a water fountain, take a sip or two.

Crunch on ice. After you finish a soft drink, eat the ice at the bottom of your cup.

Fight the flush factor. To avoid having to get up to go to the bathroom in the middle of the night, drink your last glass of water by 8:00 or 9:00 P.M.

Feeling Drained? Drink Up

If you suspect you don't drink enough water, you're not alone. "Most people are dehydrated—they drink about 25 percent less water than they need," says Dr. Kleiner.

Exercise strenuous enough to make you perspire (three consecutive sets of tennis, for example) means your body's losing water. "Weigh yourself before and after exercise to see how much weight you lose, and drink two cups of water for every pound lost," advises Dr. Kleiner. Other experts recommend that you drink one cup of water before and after exercise, and chug at least a half-cup every 15 or 20 minutes during your workout.

Seasonal changes can sap your internal water supply as well. "Our bodies lose a lot of water in the winter due to dry heat and low humidity," says Dr. Elson. "In the summer, we lose water when we perspire."

To replenish lost fluids, drink up. You can also help trap moisture in the skin by applying a moisturizer, especially in the winter, says Dr. Elson.

CHAPTER THIRTY-ONE

Lifetime Weight Control

The Right Diet for Beautiful Skin

*I*f you're a veteran dieter, you may already know that gaining and losing the same 10, 20 or more pounds is hard on your wardrobe budget—and on your general health. Some studies have found that yo-yo dieting—or weight cycling, as doctors call it—may be worse than not shedding the extra pounds at all. No less harmful is so-called crash dieting: While on these starvation diets, people often consume 1,000 calories a day or less.

But what you may not know is that weight cycling and crash diets can be murder on skin. Gaining and losing weight over and over again can cost skin its youthful firmness and elasticity. And crash diets can turn skin rough, dry and lifeless after only a few days.

The most expensive moisturizers and makeup in the world won't do a bit of good if weight cycling has left skin less taut than it could be or if a starvation diet has depleted skin of the vitamins and minerals it needs to repair itself. But you can peel away the pounds without imperiling your skin. Here's how.

Can Your Skin Make a Snappy Comeback?

No one's actually studied the effects of yo-yo dieting on skin. But generally speaking, the more body weight fluctuates, say experts, the harder it is for skin to snap back into place when the pounds come off. "It isn't good for skin to be continually stretched and released," says Barbara Gilchrest, M.D., professor and chairman of dermatology at Boston University Medical Center.

Weight cycling leads to wear and tear on collagen, the substance that helps keep skin firm and taut, says Melvin L. Elson, M.D., medical director of the Dermatology Center in Nashville and co-author of *The Good Look Book*.

"We have a fixed number of fat cells, which are situated under the top layer of skin," he explains. "When you gain weight, these cells enlarge and stretch the skin." When you shed the pounds again, says Dr. Elson, the fat cells shrink. So does your skin—hopefully.

"But suppose you keep gaining and losing weight over the years," continues Dr. Elson. "With each weight gain, the fat cells enlarge and press up against the collagen fibers, which give skin its structural support." These fibers can eventually wear out, leaving skin unable to snap back, says Dr. Elson. "Skin is like a balloon," he says. "If you keep blowing it up and letting out the air, you're eventually going to weaken it."

The yo-yo syndrome can affect skin anywhere on the body, including the hips, breasts and buttocks. But you're most likely to notice loose, sagging skin on your face and neck, says Dr. Elson. Also, gaining weight rapidly during the up phase of weight cycling can damage your skin's supply of collagen. The result: stretch marks, says Dr. Gilchrest.

The Not-So-Great Crash

While weight cycling can cost skin its firmness, crash diets can literally starve skin. "When you crash diet, you're depriving your skin, hair and nails of the nutrients they need to live," says Dr. Elson. Crash diets can also strip skin of vitamin C, which helps form collagen, and vitamin E, which helps keep cells healthy, says Jeffrey B. Blumberg, Ph.D., professor of nutrition at Tufts University in Boston.

Not surprisingly, crash diets tend to make skin look lousy, says Dr. Elson. "Cell turnover decreases, so skin begins to get coarse and dry. It won't retain moisture as well because skin cells will be less plump and less healthy. Skin may even begin to form fine lines because it can't save water as it should," says Dr. Elson.

The emotional tension that often accompanies deprivation diets can cause skin to flare, too. "The stress of struggling through a crash diet is likely to aggravate skin conditions known to be affected by stress, like acne, eczema and psoriasis," says Dr. Elson.

Almost D-Day? Safeguard Your Skin

To benefit your health and your skin, you need to avoid unhealthy weight-loss traps like weight cycling and crash diets and adopt healthier eating habits, says Michael R. Lowe, Ph.D., associate professor of clinical psychology at Hahnemann University in Philadelphia and a consultant for Weight Watchers. "The biggest mistake yo-yo dieters make is paying too little attention to their eating and exercise habits most of the time and then making too many radical changes at once when they get fed up with their weight," says Dr. Lowe.

The key, then, is to make such changes gradually. The following three-point plan is not a diet. (Consult your doctor before you begin any weight-loss diet.) But it may help you diet more healthfully—a change that could be reflected in the quality of your skin.

Plan every meal. Design your own eating schedule, suggests Dr. Lowe. "Plan your meals and snacks," he says. "Eat anything you like, but stay within your schedule." This tactic can help you set food limits even before you cut back on calories, says Dr. Lowe.

Get moving. People who stick to a regular exercise program have the best chance of keeping the pounds off permanently, says Dr. Lowe, which would end the yo-yo syndrome for good.

Lose the fat and load up on carbohydrates. The American Heart Association recommends keeping fat intake to less than 30 percent of daily calories. "Eat more grains, whole-grain bread, potatoes and pasta," says Susan M. Kleiner, R.D., Ph.D., a Seattle nutritionist and author of *The High Performance Cookbook*. "You won't have much room left for fat." You can cut even more fat, she suggests, by switching from whole to 1 percent or skim milk and from butter to fat-free margarine.

Eating more fresh fruits and vegetables and grains—without fatty sauces, dressings or butter—may help you reduce your fat intake automatically. Dr. Kleiner suggests you follow the U.S. Department of Agriculture's nutritional guidelines, which recommend 3 to 5 servings of vegetables, 2 to 4 servings of fruit and 6 to 11 servings of bread, cereal, rice and pasta a day.

CHAPTER THIRTY-TWO

Antioxidants

Can These Supervitamins Stop the Clock?

Can taking vitamins, or actually applying them to the skin, help skin look younger longer? Maybe, maybe not. Some research suggests that certain nutrients called antioxidants—first associated with reduced risks of heart disease and cancer—might also be able to slow age-related skin damage.

The antioxidant nutrients include vitamins C and E and beta-carotene, which the body converts to vitamin A. Foods rich in antioxidant nutrients include carrots, broccoli and fatty fish. Some experts believe the minerals selenium, copper and zinc have antioxidant powers as well. Antioxidants appear to delay or prevent aging and disease by destroying free radicals—unstable molecules found in the body and in the environment that attack and damage healthy cells and tissues, including those in the skin.

However, there's no conclusive proof that antioxidants can keep skin from aging. And while some dermatologists are intrigued by antioxidants' seeming ability to prevent disease, they say they aren't yet convinced that these vitamins and minerals can turn back time for the skin.

So should you eat more antioxidant-rich foods, or take antioxidant supplements, to safeguard your skin? To help you decide, here are the facts about these supervitamins.

Why Skin Ages: A Radical Theory

As mentioned elsewhere in this book, it's the cumulative effect of sun exposure—not birthdays—that damages skin most. But more and more researchers are beginning to believe that oxidation, a natural chemical reaction, may play a crucial role in causing the body—including the skin—to age.

"Oxidation is the same chemical reaction that causes iron to rust, bananas to turn brown and oil to turn rancid," explains Jeffrey B. Blumberg, Ph.D., professor of nutrition at Tufts University in Boston. Oxidation also causes reactions that eventually result in the breakdown of elastin and collagen, the materials that keep skin youthfully firm, says Dr. Kligman.

Free radicals—the by-products of oxidation that result from body functions like breathing and muscle activity—harm skin by attacking and damaging skin cells, says Dr. Blumberg. Toxins in the environment, including pollution, car exhaust, pesticides and cigarette smoke, accelerate production of free radicals, adding to the damage.

Sunlight is a potent source of free radicals, says Melvin L. Elson, M.D., medical director of the Dermatology Center in Nashville and co-author of *The Good Look Book*. While unprotected sun exposure damages skin, "it's really the free radicals that result from sun exposure that do the dirty work that we see as sun damage," notes Dr. Elson.

Antioxidants: The Toxic Avengers?

Experts agree that the ability of antioxidants to quench, or capture, free radicals may protect us from certain diseases. But the jury's still out on whether antioxidants can postpone the visible signs of aging. Says Dr. Blumberg, "There's a fair amount of experimental evidence in human cell cultures and animal studies that high doses of antioxidants may protect skin against sun damage—wrinkling and thinning skin. We also know that antioxidants play an important role in healing wounds." But he says there's just not enough evidence to prove beyond a doubt that antioxidants can help delay skin damage.

Barbara Gilchrest, M.D., professor and chairman of dermatology at Boston University Medical Center, was among a group of researchers who studied the effects of vitamin E and beta-carotene supplements on human skin exposed to ultraviolet (UV) light. She concluded that the antioxidants had "no demonstrable beneficial effect" on skin.

"In my view, the evidence that taking antioxidant vitamins by mouth or applying them to the skin has any impact on intrinsic aging or photoaging is exceedingly weak," says Dr. Gilchrest. "It's one thing to show you can prevent oxidation in a laboratory dish and another to show you can make a detectable change in the appearance or function of skin over time."

Dr. Elson disagrees. "There's not yet absolute proof that taking antioxidant supplements delays aging of the skin, decreases the risk of cancer or boosts immunity," he says. "But I believe that they do."

And the results of some experiments are encouraging. Researchers at the University of Western Ontario, for example, showed that a certain form of vitamin E, tocopherol acetate, prevented sunburn in hairless mice when applied within eight hours of exposure. Their finding suggests that this type of vitamin E could be an effective after-sun treatment. But don't use the oil from supplements on your skin. Supplements contain vitamin E in its pure state, which quickly turns rancid when exposed to air. Worse, applying pure vitamin E to the skin can actually aggravate sun damage in some people.

Want Glowing Skin? Crunch a Carrot

There's so much evidence in favor of a diet rich in antioxidants for other health problems, like heart disease, that it doesn't hurt to ensure that you consume your fair share of vitamins A, C and E. To get the Recommended Dietary Allowance (RDA) of vitamin A, is it better to eat a carrot or swallow a vitamin supplement? Most experts recommend the carrot. "There's no substitute for getting nutrients through food," says Seattle-based nutritionist Susan M. Kleiner, R.D., Ph.D., author of *The High Performance Cookbook*. "The body absorbs and assimilates them far better than in supplement form."

To feed your skin with antioxidants, eat three to five servings of vegetables and two to four servings of fruit a day, as recommended by the U.S. Department of Agriculture's Food Guide Pyramid, says Dr. Kleiner. "For vitamin C, choose at least one citrus fruit—an orange, a grapefruit—every day," says Dr. Kleiner. "And to increase your intake of beta-carotene, make sure you eat at least two orange-yellow or leafy green vegetables a day."

The RDAs for antioxidants are very small. Drinking a cup of orange juice and eating one carrot a day will give you twice the RDAs of vitamin C and beta-carotene, notes Dr. Kleiner. But you may find it harder to meet the RDA for vitamin E, especially if less than 25 percent

Munch Your Way to Beautiful Skin (Maybe)

Here are the Recommended Dietary Allowances (RDAs) for three common antioxidant nutrients, good sources of the vitamins and tips on how to maximize their benefits.

Vitamin	RDA	Sources	Tips
C	60 mg. (½ cup orange juice = 70 mg.)	→ Citrus fruits and juices → Tomatoes	→ Eat whole fruit for extra fiber. → Squeeze your own juice if possible. → Avoid juice in glass containers and heat-pasteurized juice: Light and heat destroy some C.
E	8 mg (12 IU), women; 10 mg. (15 IU), men (1 Tbsp. canola oil = 9 mg.)	→ Nuts, seeds and their oils → Fatty fish (salmon, mackerel, halibut, trout) → Wheat germ	→ Try using canola, olive or another vegetable oil in place of butter or margarine in cooking.
Beta-carotene	No established RDA; Susan M. Kleiner, R.D., Ph.D., author of *The High Performance Cookbook*, recommends 5–6 mg./day. (1 carrot = 12 mg.)	→ Orange or yellow vegetables (carrots, yams, winter squash) → Leafy green vegetables (kale, collards, spinach, broccoli)	→ Munch a bowl of prepackaged, washed and peeled baby carrots instead of popcorn while watching television.

of your daily calories come from fat, she says. If you're following a low-fat diet, "don't be afraid to add a couple of tablespoons of olive oil to your diet, or to eat some nuts or seeds," says Dr. Kleiner.

Supplements: The Formula for Safe Success

Unless you're under the care of a nutritionist or physician, meet the RDAs for antioxidants with food rather than supplements, advises Dr. Kleiner. But if for some reason you suspect you can't meet the RDAs through diet alone, take one multivitamin/mineral supplement per day, suggests Kenneth H. Neldner, M.D., professor of dermatology at Texas Tech University Health Sciences Center in Lubbock. Or take one all-in-one antioxidant vitamin supplement per day, says Dr. Kleiner.

Some researchers say that the RDAs for antioxidants are much too low and should be raised. But other experts, including Dr. Gilchrest and Dr. Neldner, say there's no evidence to support taking more than the RDAs. "People tend to think that if a little is good, a lot should be much better. But that's not always true," says Dr. Neldner.

What's more, taking vitamins can't compensate for bad skin-care habits, says Dr. Blumberg: "Antioxidants won't protect skin from excessive sun exposure, not using sunscreen or getting a sunburn."

Caution: Never take excessive amounts of vitamins A and E. These vitamins are stored in body tissue and can be toxic, says Albert M. Kligman, M.D., Ph.D. Also, excessive amounts of vitamin C can damage the kidneys.

Do Vitamin Creams Work? Here's the Rub

Can you rub away wrinkles as easily as rubbing in a moisturizer? Most dermatologists say over-the-counter creams formulated with antioxidants don't work.

Adding antioxidants to skin creams sounds reasonable enough: If taking antioxidants by mouth can help prevent age-related damage internally, then applying them directly to the skin should help prevent external damage. But experts say that most over-the-counter products don't contain enough of the vitamins to be effective. The amounts used in research experiments are much larger. What's more, vitamins are chemically unstable and tend to break down when added to cosmetics. "We don't yet have the technology to deliver enough vitamins into the skin to protect it from free-radical damage," says Dr. Elson.

There is one vitamin-based cream found to erase wrinkles and prevent new ones from forming—Retin-A, available by prescription.

See also the chapter on Retin-A (chapter 51).

PART FOUR

Quick and Easy Daily Routines for Your Skin Type

CHAPTER THIRTY-THREE

Oily Skin

Shine-Free Strategies for Beautiful Skin

*I*f you have oily skin, consider yourself blessed: The oil you bemoan now will beautify your complexion later.

"Oily skin is more resistant to sun damage, harsh treatment and wrinkles than, say, fair or dry skin," says Albert M. Kligman, M.D., Ph.D.

But while oily skin can bounce back from insult after insult, punishing your skin with harsh cleansing products to scrub away oil can leave your complexion dull and flaky. And if you have mature skin, bear in mind that your oil glands produce less oil after menopause. So continuing an oily skin-care regimen out of habit rather than necessity may be hurting rather than helping your skin.

The bottom line? Your natural oil is a built-in lubricant, a beauty oasis. So don't fight oil—control it.

Cleansing: The No-Scrub Rule

You scour your face with a harsh soap, use astringent to dry up the oil and then slather on moisturizer to ease the tightness and flaking that the astringent has left behind. That's the way to keep oily skin in line, right? Wrong: While drying soaps and alcohol-based astringents do cut oil, over time they can damage your skin. And despite what you may have heard, trying to scrub away oil is even worse. "Trying to get rid of oil by scrubbing your skin with abrasive facial pads and grainy cleansers is the worst thing you can do—it can actually stimulate your oil glands to produce more oil," says Paula A. Moynahan, M.D., attending plastic and reconstructive surgeon at Lenox Hill Hospital in New York City and St. Mary's Hospital and Waterbury Hospital in Waterbury, Connecticut.

To keep your skin at its loveliest, cleanse with soaps that have been proven to be mild. "Oil of Olay's cleansing bar and Dove are quite mild," says Dr. Kligman. If you have oily skin, avoid superfatted soaps that contain emollients like cocoa butter, lanolin or olive oil, however. While they're gentle, your complexion doesn't need the extra oil they contain.

You might also try a soap-free liquid cleanser formulated specifically for oily skin. "Liquid cleansers are the mildest of all," says Dr. Kligman. Look for a clear formula rather than a milky-white or opaque one—a sign of added moisturizers your skin doesn't need, says Wendy E. Roberts, M.D., director of dermatopathology and assistant professor of dermatology at Loma Linda University Medical Center in Loma Linda, California.

Unless you break out, avoid drying antiseptic or antibacterial cleansers, advises Dr. Roberts. And when you've found the perfect product, resist the urge to wash your face ten times a day: Like scrubbing, overcleansing can rile your oil glands into producing more oil. "Wash as little as you can—just enough to feel clean and comfortable," says Dr. Kligman.

The Harsh Truth about Astringents

Astringents—commonly formulated with alcohol and little else—remove dirt and oil, temporarily shrink pores and can give your skin a pleasant feeling of tautness. But tightness doesn't equal cleanliness: Use too much astringent on a daily basis and even the oiliest skin can flake, peel, sting or burn.

"If your skin is so oily you feel you must use an astringent, limit it to twice a day," says Dr. Moynahan. "But don't whip out the astringent every time you feel the oil pooling."

If you have oily skin, reserve astringent for wiping away oil between cleansings or during your workout. "Tuck a few astringent pads, like those made by Stridex and Sea Breeze, into your gym bag and use them during your workout to wipe away oil and perspiration—a mix that can provoke a breakout," says Marianne O'Donoghue, M.D., associate professor of dermatology at Rush Presbyterian–St. Luke's Medical Center in Chicago.

Do You Really Need to Moisturize?

Whether to use a moisturizer depends on how oily your skin is— or how much overzealous cleansing has dried out your skin.

If your complexion is only mildly oily, you can use a moisturizer with an oil-in-water emulsion under your makeup. (An oil-in-water emulsion means the moisturizer is more water than oil. To find one, look at the product's ingredient list; water should come first.) But to ease surface dryness caused by overcleansing or too much astringent, try an oil-free moisturizer. "An oil-free moisturizer will hold in your skin's own moisture or draw in moisture from the atmosphere without adding oiliness," says Dr. Moynahan.

Extremely oily skin rarely needs any type of moisturizer: "Your own oil serves as a built-in barrier to dryness," says Dr. Kligman. So don't use what you don't need: "Women have to be careful not to get tricked at cosmetics counters into buying creams and moisturizers they don't need," says Dr. O'Donoghue.

Makeup That Licks Oil Slicks

If a perpetually shiny complexion has got you down, fret not. You can find plenty of cosmetics that soak up excess oil and keep your skin fresh and beautiful.

Oil-free and water-based foundations are your best bet. They won't add extra oil to an already oily complexion, and they're a good choice if you also use a moisturizer, says Dr. Roberts. "That way, your face doesn't get a double dose of oil," she says.

Oil-blotting foundations delay shine by soaking up excess facial oil. Some oil-blotting powders, like Coty Correctives Face Powder, can even be worn in place of foundation. "Oil-blotting makeup doesn't stop your skin from producing oil, it just makes the oil invisible," says Dr. Kligman. You'll also want to use powder rather than cream blushers and—if your skin is extremely oily—powdered rather than soft pencil shadows.

To de-shine your nose and forehead during the day, try oil-blotting papers—postage-stamp-size booklets of tissue paper lightly dusted with powder. Blotting papers are quick and easy to use: You press them to oily areas and then throw them away. Look for a product called Papier Poudre (available in cosmetics stores or drugstores).

A pat or two of translucent (no-color) pressed powder compact like Cornsilk will also cut oily shine. But don't use powder more than once or twice a day: You could end up looking like you've been slapped with a chalkboard eraser!

Sun Damage? You're Not Immune

Despite what you may have heard, having oily skin doesn't protect you from the sun. "It's a myth," says Dr. Moynahan—even thick, oily skin is vulnerable to sun damage and photoaging, which causes wrinkles and rough, mottled skin. If you're worried about adding more oil to your skin, try oil-free sunscreens: They keep your skin sun-safe without adding extra shine to an already shiny complexion.

Do's and Don'ts for Oily Skin

Do ...
→ Reevaluate your skin-care routine as you get older, when oil production slows.
→ Use a mild liquid cleanser formulated for oily skin in the morning and before bed.
→ Use astringents sparingly, if at all.
→ Choose an oil-free or light oil-in-water moisturizer, if necessary.
→ Use oil-blotting or oil-free foundation and powder.
→ Use sunscreen to prevent wrinkles and other signs of photodamage.

Don't ...
→ Overdry your skin—oil is a natural defense against the elements.
→ Cleanse more than two times a day (three if you exercise).
→ Be an astringent junkie.
→ Use moisturizer if you don't need it.
→ Overuse powder to mop up oil; your skin will look chalky.

See also the chapters on blemishes (chapter 2), cleansers (chapter 22), foundation, blusher and powder (chapter 25), moisturizers (chapter 27) and sunscreen (chapter 28).

CHAPTER THIRTY-FOUR

Dry Skin

Give Your Complexion a New Glow

*I*f dry skin leads the list of your beauty woes, take heart: Your complexion may not be as dry as you think. While that tight, parched feeling can be age-related, dry skin may also be caused by a cleanser that's too harsh, a moisturizer that's not rich enough for your skin's needs or rough treatment, like overscrubbing with a grainy facial cleanser.

So before you cry dry, take a closer look at your skin-care routine: "If you have truly dry skin, you're dry everywhere—your face, your scalp, your body," says Wilma F. Bergfeld, M.D., head of clinical research and dermatopathology at the Cleveland Clinic Foundation. "And cold, dry weather just aggravates the problem."

But relief is possible: An extra-gentle cleansing routine teamed with the right moisturizer can help make even the thirstiest skin lovelier and more supple.

The Best Cleansers for Dry Skin

Dry skin tends to be thinner and less oily than other skin types, so it can't recover from harsh cleansers as easily. "It's important to find a cleanser that removes dirt and makeup thoroughly without hanging your skin out to dry," says Albert M. Kligman, M.D., Ph.D.

Signs of Dry Skin

→ Roughness to the touch
→ Flakiness, tightness
→ Occasional itchiness
→ Rare breakouts

But don't turn to soap. Many soaps, especially antibacterial or deodorant soaps, can chap dry skin, leaving it vulnerable to rashes caused by makeup or other skin-care products, explains Marianne O'Donoghue, M.D., associate professor of dermatology at Rush Presbyterian–St. Luke's Medical Center in Chicago. Your eyelids are particularly vulnerable, especially if your skin is sensitive as well as dry.

So scrap soap and opt for a soap-free cleanser instead. There are many to try, including superfatted bars (often called beauty bars) with added emollients like olive oil or lanolin, milky liquids or tissue-off cleansing creams. If your skin is severely dry, you might try Cetaphil, a cleanser that can be used without water, says Paula A. Moynahan, M.D., attending plastic and reconstructive surgeon at Lenox Hill Hospital in New York City and St. Mary's Hospital and Waterbury Hospital in Waterbury, Connecticut. "You can rinse it off it you prefer, and it's so mild just about anyone can use it," says Dr. Moynahan.

Oily cleansers, especially the tissue-off kind, can make even the driest skin sprout blemishes, however. So make sure your cleanser is labeled noncomedogenic (formulated without ingredients known to cause blemishes). But even noncomedogenic cleansers aren't guaranteed blemishproof, so "if you're breaking out after two to six weeks, try another cleanser," says Dr. Bergfeld.

Let Your Fingers Do the Washing

Your morning cleansing routine couldn't be simpler: "Just splash or mist your face with water to hydrate it," says Dr. Bergfeld.

At night, use your fingertips to gently remove makeup and dirt, says Dr. Moynahan. Don't use a washcloth or an abrasive facial pad; they're too rough for dry skin. Here's Dr. Moynahan's suggested cleansing technique.

1. If you're using a lathering cleanser, make suds in the palm of your hand, then transfer the lather to your fingertips or a disposable cotton pad.
2. Massage the cleanser into your skin, moving fingers or pad in a circular motion.
3. Rinse or tissue off the cleanser as directed on the label.
4. Gently blot your face dry with a soft towel. Never rub.
5. Apply moisturizer while your skin is still damp to seal in the moisture your skin has just absorbed.

The Best Moisturizer Is the One That Works for You

If you're like many women with dry skin, you may be moisturizing morning, noon and night in the hopes of staving off further dryness. But this strategy can backfire. Dr. O'Donoghue notes that moisturizing too often can trigger blemishes. So unless your skin is extremely dry, "moisturizing once a day, either under makeup or at night after cleansing, may be enough," she says.

Even if you prefer to moisturize more often, it's a good idea to use the lightest product that relieves the dryness. There's no need to buy a separate neck cream, says Dr. O'Donoghue. She suggests using a separate eye cream, however; they contain certain preservatives to prevent eye infections in this sensitive area.

To hydrate mildly dry skin, try a moisturizer with an oil-in-water emulsion (meaning that the product is more water than oil). These light moisturizers penetrate the skin easily and don't leave a sticky, greasy feeling behind.

Use a heavier product if your skin is moderately dry. A moisturizer with a water-in-oil emulsion (which contains more oil than water), like Eucerin, Moisturel or Nivea, will likely fit the bill. You can even mix a dab of these more solid, oil-rich moisturizers into your foundation to chap-proof your skin in cold weather.

Seriously dry skin requires an extremely heavy emollient, says Dr. Kligman. "If you have really dry skin, the best thing to use is petroleum jelly—the worse the product feels in terms of greasiness, the better it is," he says. Fortunately, you might only need to grease up at night or during the winter to protect your skin from a drying home heating system or cold- and wind-induced chapping.

If your skin is so severely dry that nothing you do seems to help, consider seeing a dermatologist, advises Dr. Kligman. She may prescribe a prescription moisturizer like Lac-Hydrin 12. There's also an outside chance that, unbeknownst to you, an underlying medical condition is at the root of your problem, in which case medical advice is the answer.

Creamy Makeup Can Quench Parched Skin

When it comes to choosing makeup for dry skin, the rule of thumb is, the creamier, the better: Oil-rich cosmetics give dry skin an extra moisture boost and can hide tiny dry lines, making dry skin look fresher and more dewy.

So if you have dry skin, choose oil-based rather than water-based foundations. (To make sure you're selecting an oil-based makeup, look for words like *hydrating, nourishing* and *moisturizing* on the product's label.) Avoid matte foundations, which dry to a nonshiny, rather than a moist, finish. Also, select creamy blushers that come in a jar or tube or the newer cream-powder blushers (many of which are formulated for dry skin). No matter how pretty the shade, powder blushers can emphasize dryness and fine lines.

For Younger-Looking Skin, Slather on the Sunscreen

Make a beeline for the sunscreen. Dry skin produces less oil than other skin types, so it's more vulnerable to sun damage, including age spots, blotches and wrinkles.

You can lessen your risk of skin damage by using a sunscreen with a sun protection factor (SPF) of at least 15 year-round and switching to an SPF 30 in the summer. You might even opt for a sunblock, which contains a physical barrier like titanium dioxide that shields skin from both ultraviolet-A light, which causes photoaging, and ultraviolet-B light, which causes sunburns and skin cancer.

You can further protect your skin by using a moisturizer with added sunscreens. Two of many are Lubriderm Lotion UV SPF 15 and Oil of Olay Daily UV Protectant Beauty Fluid SPF 15.

When Dry Skin Isn't

If your skin doesn't respond to even the greasiest moisturizers, you may have seborrheic dermatitis, an itchy, sometimes painful skin rash that may look and feel dry but is actually oily. Doctors call the condition seb derm for short. Signs of seb derm, which usually affects the scalp and occasionally the face, include redness or scaling around oily areas like your forehead, eyebrows, nose, chin and mouth.

Never use a moisturizer on seb derm. Moisturizer may be a food source for the type of yeast thought to cause the rash. Conversely, washing your hair with a dandruff shampoo twice a week may help clear up your face by reducing the oil on your scalp and face, says Dr. O'Donoghue. You can ease the redness and scaling with an over-the-counter hydrocortisone cream. But consult a dermatologist if you can't clear up the condition within a few weeks.

Do's and Don'ts for Dry Skin

Do . . .
→ Cleanse thoroughly at night to remove makeup. In the morning, simply splash your face with lukewarm water.
→ Moisturize while your skin is still damp from cleansing.
→ Slather very dry skin with the heaviest moisturizer you can tolerate.
→ Choose creamy, oil-rich makeup.
→ Prevent sun damage by using a strong sunscreen daily.

Don't . . .
→ Wash your face with soap. Choose a mild, soap-free liquid cleanser instead.
→ Scrub your face with abrasive pads, washcloths or grainy cleansers.
→ Continue to use a moisturizer that makes you break out.
→ Mistake seborrheic dermatitis for dry skin; see a dermatologist if you're not sure.

See also the chapters on dandruff and related problems (chapter 9), cleansers (chapter 22), foundation, blusher and powder (chapter 25), moisturizers (chapter 27), sunscreen (chapter 28) and oily skin (chapter 33).

CHAPTER THIRTY-FIVE

Combination Skin

Just-Right Care for (Nearly) Normal Skin

*Y*our forehead, nose and chin shine with oil; your cheeks are tight and dry. But the surest tipoff that you have combination skin is a jumble of half-used cleansers, toners and moisturizers cluttering up your bathroom shelves.

Dermatologists say combination skin is actually quite normal: We all tend to be oilier around the so-called T-zone—the forehead, nose and chin—and drier around the perimeter of the face (think of it as the U-zone). Just how oily the T-zone can be varies, of course. But combination skin can be as simple to care for as dry or oily skin—and you don't need to use a dozen different products to keep it looking its best.

In fact, you may think of combination skin as basically good, it-ain't-broke-so-don't-fix-it skin. To find out how to keep it in top condition, read on.

Cleansing: Mastering the Balancing Act

Caring for combination skin requires balancing the requirements of drier areas like the cheeks with oiliness in the T-zone, says Paula A. Moynahan, M.D., attending plastic and reconstructive surgeon at

Signs of Combination Skin

→ Oiliness in the T-zone (forehead, nose and chin)
→ Dryness on the cheeks
→ Occasional breakouts in oily areas

Lenox Hill Hospital in New York City and St. Mary's Hospital and Waterbury Hospital in Waterbury, Connecticut.

"In most women, the differences between oily and dry areas aren't major," says Dr. Moynahan. "You may have a bit more oil in the T-zone than on the rest of your face, but not at the level of all-over oily or acne-prone skin." So cleanse your T-zone as you cleanse the rest of your face, advises Dr. Moynahan, and don't break your budget on cleansers. "You don't need to use different products for different parts of your face. Women are just too busy for that," she says.

And you don't have to spring for a hodgepodge of expensive products when cleansers for combination skin can do the balancing act for you. Two of many are Neutrogena's Fresh Foaming Cleanser and Sea Breeze Daily Cleansing Wash for Normal/Combination Skin.

You can use astringent on your T-zone, says Marianne O'Donoghue, M.D., associate professor of dermatology at Rush Presbyterian–St. Luke's Medical Center in Chicago. But limit it to once a day. "Use astringents when you're sweating—when you're working out," suggests Dr. O'Donoghue. "That's when it can help stop acne."

Combination skin isn't immune to breakouts. If blemishes sprout within your T-zone, dab them with a benzoyl peroxide product after cleansing, says Wilma F. Bergfeld, M.D., head of clinical research and dermatopathology at the Cleveland Clinic Foundation. You can find benzoyl peroxide products in 2.5, 5 and 10 percent concentrations, but try the lower-strength product first.

Perspiration and oil can make your skin vulnerable to breakouts, especially when you exercise. So don't wear moisturizer or makeup to the gym, track or tennis court, blot oils and perspiration from your skin during and after exercise and freshen your T-zone with astringent towelettes.

Moisturizing to a *T*

The golden rule of moisturizing combination skin: Use a moisturizer only where you need it. The last thing you want is to make already-oily areas oilier, possibly triggering a breakout.

Moisturize the drier areas of your face with a thin lotion like Lubriderm or, if necessary, a richer cream like Nivea, especially before bed, says Albert M. Kligman, M.D., Ph.D. Your T-zone is less likely to need a moisturizer. But if you use moisturizer as a makeup prep, make sure it's oil-free.

The thin, delicate skin under your eyes may need an extra moisture boost. So choose a product specifically formulated for the eye area, advises Dr. O'Donoghue. Eye creams contain certain preservatives that keep them sterile and prevent eye infections.

No-Hassle Makeup

Most women with combination skin can use just one foundation, says Laura Geller, makeup artist and owner of Laura Geller Make-Up Studios, a cosmetics store in New York City. "If you don't use a moisturizer on your T-zone and choose a foundation formulated with just a little bit of oil, chances are you can use it over your entire face," says Geller. You may want to try a water-based foundation, which contains a small amount of oil. But if your T-zone is extremely oily, says Geller, try using an oil-free foundation, using a moisturizer on dry areas first.

Choose a powder blush, says Geller. "While your cheeks may be dry, a creamy blush may make your skin appear more oily," she says. To keep your cheeks from looking dry, says Geller, "use a blush with a low pearl finish, but not one that's highly frosted."

Use a cream-formula lipstick to keep lips smooth and moist, says Geller. "Avoid frosted formulas to deflect attention away from an oily T-zone." For the same reason, avoid frosted eye shadows and choose matte finishes, she says.

Don't Skimp on Sunscreen

There's no doubt about it: Using sunscreen can keep wrinkles and other sun-related skin damage (roughness, mottling, age spots) at bay. So slather on a generous dollop of sunscreen (or an oil-free mois-

turizer with added sunscreen) every day. Most dermatologists recommend using a sunscreen with a sun protection factor (SPF) of 15
or higher.

Do's and Don'ts for Combination Skin

Do...
- → Choose cleansers for combination skin; they're formulated to be
  gentle on dry spots, tougher on the T-zone.
- → Apply products only where you need them—moisturizer only
  on dry areas, benzoyl peroxide products right on blemishes.
- → Smooth on a sunscreen with SPF 15 or a moisturizer or founda-
  tion with built-in sunscreen protection every day.
- → Cleanse oils and perspiration from skin during and after exercise.

Don't...
- → Use two kinds of cleanser or moisturizer on different parts of
  your face; seek out products formulated for combination skin.
- → Use balancing lotions; they neither endow dry areas with mois-
  ture nor reduce the amount of oil your oil glands produce.
- → Apply moisturizer or makeup before working out.
- → Forget to wear sunscreen.

See also the chapters on blemishes (chapter 2), dandruff and related
problems (chapter 9), cleansers (chapter 22), foundation, blusher and
powder (chapter 25), moisturizers (chapter 27), sunscreen (chapter
28) and oily skin (chapter 33).

CHAPTER THIRTY-SIX

Fair Skin

Keeping an "English Rose" Complexion in Bloom

*I*f fair skin could talk, it would probably cry, "Ouch!" That's because even the loveliest peaches-and-cream complexion can be downright temperamental.

Fair skin takes everything personally—harsh soaps, hot water, cosmetic ingredients. Wind and cold often turn its milky whiteness to angry red splotches, and the sun burns it more easily, leading to quicker, deeper sun damage and premature wrinkling.

So if you have fair skin, the heart of your skin-care regimen is a good defense. "Fair skin is often sensitive, and you have to treat it more carefully," says Paula A. Moynahan, M.D., attending plastic and reconstructive surgeon at Lenox Hill Hospital in New York City and St. Mary's Hospital and Waterbury Hospital in Waterbury, Connecticut.

But you can give your fair skin the pampering it needs. Cleansers and moisturizers formulated for delicate skin, makeup with added sun protection and strong sunscreens can all work together to keep your skin calm, smooth and beautiful.

Caution! Cleanse with Care

Fair skin needs a gentle cleanser, and a soap-free, detergent-based liquid cleanser like Cetaphil or Moisturel Sensitive Skin Cleanser usually fits the bill. But don't lather up more than once a day. "Even mild cleansers can irritate your skin if you use them too often," says Albert M. Kligman, M.D., Ph.D.

So keep your cleansing routine as basic as your cleanser. In the morning, a splash of lukewarm water and a gentle blotting with a soft towel is often all the cleansing fair skin needs. "Skin doesn't give a damn if it's dirty or not!" says Dr. Kligman. At night, remove your makeup with your liquid cleanser. "Apply the cleanser with your fingertips—no washcloths or abrasives—and rinse with warm, not hot, water," says Dr. Kligman.

As unlikely as it sounds, fair skin can sometimes be oily. But steer clear of harsh soaps and astringents. "Oily fair skin is usually so sensitive that you can't use strong degreasers," explains Marianne O'Donoghue, M.D., associate professor of dermatology at Rush Presbyterian–St. Luke's Medical Center in Chicago. Instead, opt for cleansers formulated for normal to oily skin.

When It Comes to Moisturizers, Get Rich Quick

If your skin is dry, you can help keep it supple by moisturizing day and night—literally. By day, try a moisturizer formulated with an alpha hydroxy acid (AHA) like glycolic acid, suggest the experts. (AHAs, found in many moisturizers, including Avon's Anew, are mild fruit acids derived from foods like milk, apples and sugar cane.) "AHAs help skin retain moisture, so they're helpful if you have a dry complexion," says Dr. Moynahan.

As mild as they are, AHAs can cause some people's skin to sting. So before you apply the product to your face, advises Dr. O'Donoghue, test it by rubbing it into the crook of your arm for three nights in a row. "If the product doesn't irritate your arm, it's not likely to irritate your face," she says.

At night, use a rich, oil-based moisturizer like Eucerin, Moisturel or Nivea Creme or—Dr. Kligman's choice—petroleum jelly. Avoid lotions, which are primarily water and usually too thin to deliver the moisture your skin really needs, says Dr. Kligman. If you happen to have fair, oily skin, consider skipping a moisturizer altogether, says Dr. O'Donoghue. "If you have oily skin, you don't need one."

But whether your skin is oily or dry, fair skin is susceptible to lines and wrinkles. And despite what the ads for many over-the-counter wrinkle creams suggest, these products can't eliminate fine lines or wrinkles. For serious wrinkle relief, consider trying Retin-A (topical tretinoin). Available only by prescription, this vitamin A–based cream is the best wrinkle fighter barring cosmetic surgery (see below).

Makeup That Won't Rile Your Skin

If you have fair skin, you can make the most of your milky complexion by choosing the right type and shades of makeup.

If your skin is dry, use an oil-rich foundation, says Laura Geller, makeup artist and owner of Laura Geller Make-Up Studios, a cosmetics store in New York City. "Look for the word *luminesse* on the bottle," she suggests. "A pearlescent foundation creates a sparkle on the skin that can make your complexion look more dewy." If your skin tends to be dry and sensitive, avoid foundations that contain mineral oil, alcohol and fragrance. Avoid powdered blushers, which can make dry skin look drier; stick to creamy blushers instead. Oily fair skin can benefit from oil-blotting foundations and powders that absorb oil as it surfaces and powdered blushers. Creamy blushers tend to slip and streak on oily skin.

If you're like many fair-skinned women, your skin has a pink undertone, which is most flattered by foundations in shades of clear beige, light porcelain or alabaster, says Geller. A pink-based foundation can help brighten mature skin, especially if it tends to be sallow, says Geller. When it comes to blusher, fair skin looks lovely in a soft, cool pink. "Avoid shades of orange or terra-cotta," advises Geller. As for lipstick, choose soft, muted shades of rose and peach and avoid blue-based shades of red, like ruby or fuchsia, says Geller.

Among the most flattering shades of eyeliner for fair skin are neutral hues like taupe, charcoal and moss green. If your skin is so fair you see blue veins beneath your eyelids, prep your lids with an eye fixative, suggests Geller. "This product works much like a concealer," she says.

Sunscreen: Fair Skin's All-Weather Friend

You probably already know your skin can sizzle even on a cloudy day in March. "Fair skin doesn't have the natural melanin protection deeper skin tones have," says Dr. Moynahan. This lack of melanin—the substance that gives skin its pigment and protects it against ultraviolet light—makes fair skin extremely vulnerable to sun damage like wrinkles, roughness and blotches. Worse, fair skin is at increased risk for skin cancer.

Fortunately, it's never too late to protect your skin from the sun and undo the damage it's already sustained. "If you use a sunscreen every day, your skin will have an opportunity to renew itself and to heal," says Dr. Moynahan.

So start slathering on a sunscreen or sunblock with a sun protection factor (SPF) of at least 15 every day—even in the winter. During the summer or when you're vacationing in sunny climates, up the SPF to 25 or 30. "It's important that you use the higher SPF because your skin is a lot more vulnerable," says Dr. O'Donoghue. Whatever SPF you use, apply sunscreen 20 to 30 minutes before going out to let it soak into your skin.

If you yearn for a sun-kissed glow, self-tanners can give you a convincing artificial tan without your risking a burn. Choose the products formulated specifically for fair skin; they'll give your complexion a pretty hint of tan rather than an overbearing shade of mahogany.

If Your Fair Skin Needs Help . . .

Just as fair skin is more vulnerable to sun damage, it's more likely to show premature lines and wrinkles. A dermatologist can prescribe a variety of products to keep your skin looking younger, longer. For example, Retin-A, the prescription-only vitamin A cream, encourages cell turnover, sloughing away dead skin cells and exposing the newer, fresher skin underneath. What's more, fair skin is the ideal type for a facial peel, a nonsurgical procedure that can eliminate many of the signs of sun damage, including rough skin and wrinkles.

Fair skin is also susceptible to rosacea (pronounced ro-ZAY-shuh), a skin condition that can mimic common acne's pimples and is often called adult acne. The symptoms of rosacea include frequent flushing and blushing, the appearance of dilated blood vessels along the sides of the nose and on the cheeks and blemishes (not blackheads) that resemble common acne.

Instead of helping to eliminate pimples, over-the-counter acne medications like benzoyl peroxide can aggravate rosacea. So if you have fair skin and start seeing blemishes you've never seen before, consult a dermatologist.

Do's and Don'ts for Fair Skin

Do ...

→ Cleanse as little as possible; use a soap-free, mild liquid cleanser.

→ Moisturize with as oily a product as your skin can tolerate.

→ Wear oil-rich foundations and creamy blushers.

→ Apply an SPF 15 sunscreen or sunblock daily. Use a product with an SPF of 25 or 30 during the summer.

→ Ask your dermatologist about moisturizers formulated with alpha hydroxy acids, Retin-A and other prescription-only options to reverse sun damage and zap fine lines and wrinkles.

Don't ...

→ Irritate your delicate skin by using abrasive facial pads, astringents or other alcohol-based skin-care products.

→ Use thin lotions; most don't contain enough oil to keep skin lubricated.

→ Waste time and money on over-the-counter creams that claim they can eliminate wrinkles.

→ Self-treat sudden blemishes; you may have rosacea.

See also the chapters on blemishes (chapter 2), cleansers (chapter 22), foundation, blusher and powder (chapter 25), moisturizers (chapter 27), sunscreen (chapter 28), wrinkle creams (chapter 29), oily skin (chapter 33), dry skin (chapter 34) and chemical peels (chapter 45).

CHAPTER THIRTY-SEVEN

Ruddy Skin

Strategies for a Sensitive Complexion

Ruddy skin—that is, a predominantly red or pink complexion—has much in common with fair skin. Both tend to be dry, sensitive and prone to sun damage. And like fair-skinned folks, people with ruddy skin are more likely to develop rosacea (pronounced ro-ZAY-shuh), a chronic but treatable condition that commonly affects the skin of people of Northern European descent.

It's possible to have a ruddy complexion without developing rosacea. "But whether you have plain ruddy skin or rosacea, a gentle skin-care routine will help keep your complexion calm," says Jonathan K. Wilkin, M.D., professor of medicine and pharmacology at Ohio State University Medical Center in Columbus.

The Best Routine for Ruddy Skin

These tips can help keep your complexion at its loveliest.

Use a gentle soap. If your skin isn't excessively dry, choose a soap without added emollients, like Basis, says Dr. Wilkin. You may also try Oil of Olay Foaming Face Wash or Cetaphil. If your skin is very dry, opt for a soap with added emollients, like Dove, says Dr. Wilkin.

Above all, avoid antibacterial and deodorant soaps. "They can irritate your skin," says Dr. Wilkin.

The right way to wash. If you have ruddy skin, avoid abrasive facial pads or washcloths—they're tough on your complexion. Rather, massage your cleanser into your skin with your fingertips, then rinse well with plenty of lukewarm water. Cleanser residue can cause irritation. Then gently blot your face dry with a thick cotton towel.

Nix alcohol-based products. If your ruddy skin is normal or dry, avoid toners or astringents, says Paula A. Moynahan, M.D., attending plastic and reconstructive surgeon at Lenox Hill Hospital in New York City and at St. Mary's Hospital and Waterbury Hospital in Waterbury, Connecticut. But if you have oily skin or combination skin, with an oily forehead, nose and chin (the so-called T-zone), and feel you must use one of these products, opt for an alcohol-free toner.

Moisturize if you must. Says Dr. Wilkin, "The perception is that people of Northern European descent have drier skin. But ruddy skin can be oily or dry." Your T-zone may produce enough oil that you don't need to use a moisturizer in this area, says Dr. Wilkin. "But with ruddy skin, it's often necessary to moisturize the cheeks," he says.

On Red Alert? Makeup Can Help

The right shade of foundation can help camouflage mild ruddiness, says Laura Geller, makeup artist and owner of Laura Geller Make-Up Studios, a cosmetics store in New York City. "Choose a foundation with a soft yellow undertone, like fawn," she advises. Avoid cool shades of foundation, like a blue-based pink. Also, "don't use a shade that's so different from your own skin tone that it's obvious you're trying to hide the ruddiness," says Geller.

To help minimize very ruddy skin, wear a green-tinted underbase, a corrective concealer, under your foundation, suggests Dr. Wilkin. Don't worry: A green underbase won't make your skin appear green. It will neutralize the red. You can find green concealers at some drugstores and most department store beauty counters. Dr. Wilkin recommends Shiseido's Controlling Green. Other cosmetics companies make green-tinted concealers as well.

As for blusher, ruddy skin looks lovely in a soft, pale pink, says Geller. For a naturally bronzed look, try shades of terra-cotta. But avoid fuchsia, coral or orange blushers. On lips, soft, warm shades like light copper will most flatter your skin tone. Avoid blue-based shades, like fuchsia, or hues with a lot of red, like berry and brick.

On eyes, "try yellow-golds, earth tones without a red base, even pinks," says Geller. But again, avoid shades of blue. She also suggests that women with ruddy skin prime their lids with an eye fixative before applying eye shadow. "A fixative will block out ruddiness and help shadow stay put," says Geller.

Now Hear This: Screen Out Sun Damage

If you have ruddy skin, it's vital to protect your skin from the sun, say experts. "Generally, ruddy skin contains less pigment and is more prone to sun damage, including premature wrinkling and skin cancer," says Dr. Moynahan. "People with ruddy skin also develop broken capillaries more easily, which can lead to even more ruddiness."

To afford your skin the best protection from solar assault, smooth on a sunscreen or sunblock with a sun protection factor (SPF) of at least 15 every time you leave the house. Dr. Wilkin recommends gentle products formulated for children, like Johnson & Johnson No More Tears or Hawaiian Tropic Baby Faces. Steer clear of alcohol-based gel sunscreens that can sting your skin and aggravate ruddiness.

If unprotected sun exposure has left you with rough, red, blotchy skin, consult a dermatologist. She can prescribe a skin-care program to rejuvenate your complexion.

Do's and Don'ts for Ruddy Skin

Do . . .

→ Use a mild cleanser.
→ Wear shades of makeup that can help downplay ruddiness.
→ Camouflage extreme ruddiness by using a green underbase.
→ Apply a sunscreen with an SPF of 15 or above every day.
→ See a dermatologist if you suspect rosacea.

Don't . . .

→ Cleanse skin with abrasive products.
→ Use astringents and toners. If you feel you must use these products, opt for an alcohol-free toner.
→ Moisturize your T-zone if it's oily.
→ Forget to use sunscreen every time you go outdoors.

See also the chapters on cleansers (chapter 22), concealers (chapter 23), moisturizers (chapter 27) and sunscreen (chapter 28).

CHAPTER THIRTY-EIGHT

Olive Skin

Keeping "Good" Skin at Its Best

*I*f you're dark-haired, dark-eyed and of Mediterranean descent, you most likely have olive skin. And if you do possess this distinctive coloring (a darker Caucasian skin with a gold undertone), your skin has built-in properties that, with the right care, can keep it looking younger longer.

"Olive skin is thicker, oilier and more resistant to sun damage than lighter skin. It's a better barrier," says Albert M. Kligman, M.D., Ph.D.

Olive skin isn't perfect, of course. It's often oily and occasionally sprouts a blemish. Less often, olive skin is dry and flaky with an ashen cast or dry along the cheeks and oily across the forehead, nose and chin (so-called combination skin).

Most often, however, olive skin is good skin that resists wrinkling and sun damage and glows in virtually any shade of makeup. But even people blessed with olive skin need to be vigilant about its care. Here's how.

Olive's Oil: More a Blessing than a Curse

Many olive-complexioned women, frustrated by their skin's oily shine, try to scour away excess oil with harsh soaps, astringents and gritty facial scrubs. But overscrubbing won't dry up the oil: It may even rile your oil glands into producing more.

What's more, the oil you bemoan is what keeps your complexion soft and smooth. To maintain your skin's natural suppleness, wash in the morning and before bed with a gentle soap-free cleanser, says Marianne O'Donoghue, M.D., associate professor of dermatology at Rush Presbyterian–St. Luke's Medical Center in Chicago. (You may try Cetaphil or Neutrogena Liquid Cleansing Formula.)

Avoid overusing astringents, says Dr. O'Donoghue. The alcohol they contain can turn your complexion dull, dry and flaky. If you feel you must use astringent, choose a product formulated for sensitive skin (like Clean and Clear Sensitive Skin Astringent), which contains less alcohol.

Occasionally, olive skin may erupt in a blemish or two. If that happens, says Wendy E. Roberts, M.D., director of dermatopathology and assistant professor of dermatology at Loma Linda University Medical Center in California, don't try to scrub them away; simply spot-treat them with a 2.5 percent benzoyl peroxide product, available in drugstores.

Why You May Not Need to Moisturize

Very oily skin generally doesn't need a moisturizer, says Dr. O'Donoghue. But if your skin is only mildly oily, a light-textured, oil-free moisturizer can help your makeup glide on more smoothly without triggering a breakout.

The darker your skin, the duller it will look if it's dry. "Darker olive skin tends to flake and become ashy, and women with this type of complexion usually overmoisturize to correct the problem," says Wilma F. Bergfeld, M.D., head of clinical research and dermatopathology at the Cleveland Clinic Foundation. The result: dry, flaky skin with pimples.

Using a noncomedogenic moisturizer can ease dryness without causing blemishes, says Dr. Bergfeld. Noncomedogenic means the product doesn't contain ingredients known to clog pores.

Compliment Your Coloring

Because olive skin can be sallow or ashen, oily or dry, you need to choose makeup to match your skin type and even out your skin tone.

If you have oily skin, choose oil-free or water-based foundations and powdered blushers, and blot shine throughout the day with translucent pressed powder or oil-blotting papers (available in beauty supply stores), says Laura Geller, makeup artist and owner of Laura Geller Make-Up Studios, a cosmetics store in New York City. Give dry skin a moister, dewier look with oil-based foundations and creamy blushers.

To cool down your skin's warm yellow undertone, choose tawny or honey beige foundations, says Geller. "These shades even out the pigment of olive skin and make it less sallow," she says. Further flatter your coloring with cheek and lip colors in shades of pink or pink-red, peach, orange-based reds and browns. "Avoid any shade of coral—it can emphasize the yellow in your skin," says Geller.

Also, play up your eyes: Unlike fair- or ruddy-skinned women, olive-skinned women can wear dramatic shades of eye shadow, including emerald green, chestnut brown and matte gold as well as neutral shades like tans, browns and grays.

Sunproof Skin Still Needs Sunscreen

Make no mistake about it: While olive skin rarely burns, it's not immune to sun damage. Moreover, baking to a golden brown tan is just as bad for your skin as sustaining a sunburn. The damage just takes longer to show up. So like anyone else, women with olive complexions need to boost their skin's natural resistance to photodamage by using a sunscreen with a sun protection factor (SPF) of at least 15 year-round.

Choose an oil-free sunscreen if you have oily skin and creamier sunscreens if your skin is dry, advises Dr. O'Donoghue.

Erase Dark Circles and Look Years Younger

Many olive-skinned women complain about undereye circles. The result of too much melanin, or pigment, under the eyes, dark circles are usually hereditary (if your parents have them, chances are you will, too) and can debut as early as your twenties. Unfortunately, dark circles can also make you look years older.

You can easily camouflage undereye circles by stroking on a concealer that's no more than one shade lighter than your foundation. But to erase dark circles permanently, consider getting a chemical peel, suggests Elliot Jacobs, M.D., attending surgeon at New York Eye and Ear Infirmary and Cabrini Medical Center and a plastic surgeon in New York City. This is an in-office procedure in which a cosmetic surgeon or dermatologist uses the medium-strength trichloroacetic acid (TCA) or a stronger chemical called phenol to peel away the excess pigment, says Dr. Jacobs.

The phenol peel can leave a noticeable line of demarcation under your eyes, however, says Paula A. Moynahan, M.D., attending plastic and reconstructive surgeon at Lenox Hill Hospital in New York City and St. Mary's Hospital and Waterbury Hospital in Waterbury, Connecticut. To avoid this risk, "it may be safer to repeat a TCA peel two or three times," says Dr. Moynahan.

Also, don't go to a salon for an undereye peel. Medium and deep peels are best left to a doctor.

Do's and Don'ts for Olive Skin

Do . . .

→ Follow the skin-care routine that suits your skin type—oily, dry or combination.

→ Use oil-free foundations and powdered blushers on oily skin, oil-based makeup and creamy blushers if your complexion is dry.

→ Use makeup shades that flatter your complexion.

→ Prevent photoaging by wearing an SPF 15 sunscreen year-round.

→ Camouflage dark circles with a concealer or consider a chemical peel to get rid of circles for good.

Don't . . .

→ Take your good skin for granted. It still needs care to look its best.

→ Overuse astringents. They can leave your skin dull and flaky.

→ Use a heavier moisturizer than your skin needs. It could trigger breakouts.

→ Treat dark circles with a salon peel. It's safer to let a dermatologist treat them.

See also the chapters on blemishes (chapter 2), cleansers (chapter 22), concealers (chapter 23), foundation, blusher and powder (chapter 25), moisturizers (chapter 27), sunscreen (chapter 28), oily skin (chapter 33), dry skin (chapter 34), combination skin (chapter 35), acne-prone skin (chapter 42) and chemical peels (chapter 45).

CHAPTER THIRTY-NINE

Black Skin

Expert Advice for a Clear and Lustrous Complexion

All black skin is not alike. Tones range from very light to very dark, from honey to ebony, from even pigmentation to uneven. And no matter what you may have heard or read, not all black skin is oily. So no one skin-care routine or foundation is right for all black women.

And whether your skin is dark- or light-toned, dry or oily, one tendency is universal: Unprotected exposure to the sun accentuates changes in pigment. So contrary to what many people believe, individuals with black skin cannot spend time in the sun with impunity.

Whether or not you're exposed to the sun, black skin may be susceptible to random deposits of pigment, called melasma, or irregular loss of pigment, called vitiligo.

Foundation can help even out your complexion. But there's more to black skin care than selecting the right shade of makeup. At the very least, correct cleansing and ultraviolet protection are vital to a youthful, flawless complexion. And if you happen to develop a pigmentation problem, options are available to help keep your skin looking its best.

Most important, black women need to find a dermatologist with expertise in treating black skin, especially if they are considering cosmetic procedures that may alter their skin's pigmentation.

Black Skin Can Be Dry, Oily or Both

Strictly speaking, *black skin* designates skin tone, not skin type. "Black women can have dry, oily or combination skin," says Wendy E. Roberts, M.D., director of dermatopathology and assistant professor of dermatology at Loma Linda University Medical Center in California. Dr. Roberts sees a higher-than-average number of black women in her practice, enhancing her expertise in this area.

If your skin is oily, use a soap-free cleanser that's formulated for oily skin, says Harold E. Pierce, Jr., M.D., dermatologist and cosmetic surgeon at the Pierce Cosmetic Surgery Center in Philadelphia and professor emeritus of dermatologic cosmetic surgery at Howard University in Washington, D.C. You may try Flori Roberts Optima Gel Cleanser, for example. You should avoid true soap, however. It can eventually dry and irritate even the oiliest skin, says Dr. Pierce.

If you have dry skin, "use a mild, soap-free cleanser at night," says Dr. Roberts. In the morning, she suggests, splash your face with warm water, blot dry and apply your moisturizer while your skin is still damp.

Renew Dry, Flaky Skin's Luster with a Supermoisturizer

"If you have oily skin, you absolutely don't need a moisturizer," says Dr. Pierce. But if you like using a moisturizer as a makeup base, opt for an oil-free, noncomedogenic lotion (formulated without ingredients known to cause blemishes). "You can also hydrate mildly dry skin with an oil-free moisturizer," says Dr. Pierce.

If your skin is so dry that it peels and flakes, giving your black complexion an ashen cast, opt for a moisturizer formulated with an alpha hydroxy acid (AHA) like glycolic or lactic acid, suggests Dr. Roberts. Many dermatologists consider AHAs—derived from natural substances like fruit, milk and sugar cane—to be excellent moisturizers.

Dr. Roberts recommends Eucerin Plus Alpha Hydroxy Moisture Lotion. "It's a great over-the-counter emollient," she says. "Use it once or twice a day, and dampen your skin with water before you apply it." You may want to use a heavier moisturizer like Eucerin Creme at night, she says.

Treat Blemishes with Care—Or a Doctor's Help

For the occasional blemish, use a 2.5 percent concentration of an over-the-counter benzoyl peroxide product, says Dr. Roberts. Don't use the 5 or 10 percent concentrations, she says, because benzoyl peroxide can leave a white spot (hypopigmentation) or a dark spot (hyperpigmentation) where the blemish used to be. Don't squeeze a blemish or a blackhead, either. "You can get hyperpigmentation and scarring," says Dr. Roberts.

If you get more than an occasional pimple, consult a dermatologist, says Dr. Pierce. Black skin tends to scar or develop hyperpigmentation if acne becomes inflamed. "You can help prevent these problems by getting early treatment," he advises.

For severe acne, Dr. Pierce often prescribes benzoyl peroxide products in tandem with a topical (applied to the skin) antibiotic called erythromycin. Your dermatologist may also prescribe the oral drug Accutane (isotretinoin), which virtually shuts down oil production. This drug can have serious side effects, however, such as peeling skin, irritated eyelids and inflamed lips.

Selecting Cosmetics:
The Right Shades for Your Skin Tone

If you're African American, you need to choose makeup shades that match your underlying skin tone—usually yellow (for lighter black skin), orange (for mahogany-toned skin) or blue-red (for very dark skin).

If you have lighter black skin, choose a foundation with a golden undertone, says Laura Geller, makeup artist and owner of Laura Geller Make-Up Studios, a cosmetics store in New York City. She suggests shades of bronze, sun gold and terra-cotta—"any sun-kissed color," she says. Lighter skin tones are flattered by orange-based shades of blusher and lip colors in shades of copper, bronze, berry-brown and terra-cotta. If your skin is a rich shade of mahogany, try foundations in warm shades with yellow undertones and blushers and lipsticks in shades of rust, copper or cinnamon.

Very dark skin generally has a blue-red undertone and may appear ashen, says Geller. "Stay away from foundation shades that contain too much pink," advises Geller. "The warmer the shade, the better." You'll flatter your skin tone with blushers and lipsticks in very bright shades of salmon, hot pink and fuchsia.

How to Choose a Qualified Dermatologist

To find a dermatologist or cosmetic surgeon with expertise in treating black skin, "look for a dermatologist who trained in an area with a large population of people of color," advises Wendy E. Roberts, M.D., director of dermatopathology and assistant professor of dermatology at Loma Linda University Medical Center in California. "You should be able to find dermatologists experienced in the treatment of black skin in every major city."

Also, check a dermatologist's credentials, says Dr. Roberts. "Be sure she knows exactly how your skin should be handled—good advice no matter what color your skin and what procedure you're interested in," she says. Harold E. Pierce, Jr., M.D., professor emeritus of dermatologic cosmetic surgery at Howard University in Washington, D.C., and dermatologist and cosmetic surgeon at the Pierce Cosmetic Surgery Center in Philadelphia, suggests that you ask if the dermatologist belongs to the American Society for Dermatologic Surgery or the American Academy of Cosmetic Surgery, especially if you're considering procedures like dermabrasion or facial peels.

See also the chapters on collagen injections and other filler techniques (chapter 46) and cosmetic surgery (chapter 47).

Flori Roberts, Fashion Fair and supermodel Iman's makeup line make cosmetics specifically for black women. Many other cosmetics companies have introduced cosmetic lines especially for black skin, including Avon's Tones of Beauty, Cover Girl's Fresh Complexion and Maybelline's Shades of You.

Banish Blotches with Strong Sun Protection

No doubt about it: Black skin can and does burn. So using a sunscreen is an important part of your skin-care routine: "We all need to wear sunscreen, including people of color," says Dr. Roberts.

Wearing sun protection also helps prevent your skin from turning blotchy. "For years, black people were told, 'You don't burn, you don't tan, you don't have to worry.' That's just not true," says Dr. Pierce. To show just how unprotected sun exposure affects black skin, he has people compare the color of the skin on their face to the backs of their hands, then to their chest. "Many people don't realize their skin is three or four different shades," he says.

To prevent blotching, wear either a true sunscreen or a moisturizer or foundation with a high sun protection factor (SPF). "In the northeast, you can get away with SPF 11 to 13, like Clinique's City Block. Go for a higher SPF in sunnier zones," says Dr. Roberts. Dr. Pierce recommends wearing SPF 17 to 24. "You can't overdo sunscreen," he says. If your skin is seriously mottled, an experienced dermatologist may be able to recommend a program of hydroquinone (a skin-bleaching agent) and glycolic acid products, says Dr. Pierce.

Keloids: A Special Concern

Black skin is prone to keloids—hard, raised scars, often found on the face and neck, that can develop after trauma to the skin, including cuts, burns, severe acne and surgery. So-called spontaneous keloids can also pop up for no reason at all.

You can minimize your chances of developing keloids by avoiding trauma to the skin, particularly on the chin, says Dr. Roberts: "Constant tweezing can cause scarring, which may lead to keloid formation," she says, especially if a hair becomes ingrown. So clip unwanted chin hairs or have a qualified electrolysist remove them. Piercing the ears can also trigger keloid growth, says Dr. Pierce. "I don't encourage black people to get their ears pierced, but I would rather a doctor pierce their ears than have them go to a jewelry store in the mall," says Dr. Pierce.

Dermatologists treat keloids with acid, freezing, burning, dermabrasion and laser treatment. The latest keloid treatment is a dressing called Silastic gel sheeting, which is cut to the shape of the keloid and helps soften and flatten it. "We don't know exactly why it works, but it's the biggest advance seen in keloid treatment in the 40 years I've been practicing," says Dr. Pierce.

Even so, there's more than a 50 percent chance that a keloid will recur within seven to nine months, says Dr. Pierce. In that case, a dermatologist may prescribe injections of steroids or interferon, he says.

A Facial Peel Can Help Smooth Pigment Problems

"For years, black patients were told they couldn't correct pigment problems like melasma with cosmetic procedures like chemical peels," says Dr. Pierce. But according to Dr. Pierce, black skin can undergo procedures like a medium-strength trichloroacetic acid (TCA) peel if skin is pretreated with prescription products like Retin-A cream, alpha hydroxy acids, hydroquinone and sunscreen.

Your dermatologist may prescribe a regimen of sunblocks, AHA products and Retin-A (topical tretinoin) for four to six weeks before the peel, says Dr. Pierce. Midway through this procedure, skin looks worse rather than better, he says. "The TCA peel is an aggressive treatment and you have to persevere, but it works with predictable results," he says.

Caution: If you're African American, there's a chance that undergoing certain cosmetic procedures can cause keloids, says Dr. Pierce. So tell your dermatologist whether you or anyone in your family has a history of keloids before undergoing the procedure.

If You Have Vitiligo . . .

Vitiligo is an autoimmune disease that causes the skin to lose some of its pigment, also known as hypopigmentation (loss of pigment) of the skin. You can conceal a mild case of vitiligo with camouflage products like Dermablend, Covermark or Fashion Fair's Cover Tone Concealing Creme, which is made especially for covering vitiligo.

If vitiligo is severe, says Dr. Pierce, a dermatologist can either repigment the sections of lightened skin or depigment the rest of the skin. Both treatments are long-term and may take between 18 months and two years to complete, he says.

Darkening affected skin, usually with psoralens and ultraviolet-A (PUVA) therapy, is commonly suggested if vitiligo affects less than 20 percent of the skin. People who undergo either treatment need to use a full-spectrum sunscreen to prevent sun damage from both ultraviolet-A and ultraviolet-B rays, says Dr. Pierce. If pigment loss occurs on more than 65 percent of the body, "it's simpler to remove the rest of the pigment than to restore the original color," says Dr. Pierce. Depigmentation is usually performed with monobenzyl ether of hydroquinone, a powerful bleaching agent. "But depigmentation may impact on a person's life more than she thinks, so it deserves serious thought," says Dr. Roberts.

Do's and Don'ts for Black Skin

Do ...

→ Follow the skin-care routine suited to your skin type—oily, dry or combination.

→ Wear foundation that matches your particular skin tone.

→ See a dermatologist early if you get more than the occasional pimple. Acne can leave scars if left untreated.

→ Wear sunscreen or sunblock daily: Black skin does burn.

→ Seek a dermatologist experienced in treating black skin, especially if you're considering cosmetic surgery.

Don't ...

→ Cleanse more than once a day if your skin is dry, twice a day if it's oily.

→ Squeeze blackheads and blemishes. You may replace the blemish with a permanent dark spot.

→ Try to alter your skin tone with makeup. Use the right shade for your complexion.

→ Tweeze hairs on your chin; it may encourage a keloid. Clip hairs instead.

See also the chapters on blemishes (chapter 2), cleansers (chapter 22), concealers (chapter 23), foundation, blusher and powder (chapter 25), moisturizers (chapter 27), sunscreen (chapter 28), oily skin (chapter 33), dry skin (chapter 34), chemical peels (chapter 35), dermabrasion (chapter 48) and Retin-A (chapter 51).

CHAPTER FORTY

Mature Skin

De-aging Strategies for More Radiant Skin

*G*ood news: With the right care, skin that's late-thirtysomething, forty-something or even beyond can look more youthful. Even better, much of the damage we associate with aging skin—roughness, blotches, brown spots, wrinkling—is caused not by the passing of the years but by unprotected exposure to the sun. Translation: A lot of age-related skin damage is preventable.

As you approach midlife, your skin-care routine should center on preventing further sun damage and replenishing the moisture young skin has naturally. But it's also wise to rethink skin-care habits you've been following for years: You may need to replace an oily-skin routine with one for dry skin or intensify the dry-skin routine you already follow.

As you'll see, gentle care, a daily dose of sunscreen and the right makeup can go a long way toward restoring a woman's youthful appearance. And if you so desire, a dermatologist can offer even more rejuvenating skin treatments.

The Three-Step Formula for Younger-Looking Skin

No need to buy expensive products that may not live up to their promises. Following these few simple steps can help keep your complexion fresh and lovely.

Cleanse gently. If your formerly oily skin now feels a little dry, switch from a soap, which can be harsh, to a gentle soap-free cleanser formulated for dry skin. Try superfatted bars (sometimes called beauty bars) like Dove or soap-free liquid cleansers for dry skin. If your skin is extremely dry, try a tissue-off cleansing cream—the oiliest cleanser of all.

Uncover fresh skin. Exfoliating, or sloughing off dull, dead cells from the surface of your skin, reveals the new, fresh skin beneath. The best way to exfoliate mature skin, say experts, is with Retin-A (topical tretinoin), the prescription vitamin A cream that unglues dead surface skin cells and stimulates the skin's production of collagen, the stuff that keeps skin firm and supple. (More on Retin-A later.)

Never exfoliate with abrasive pads or grainy cleansers, says Wilma F. Bergfeld, M.D., head of clinical research and dermatopathology at the Cleveland Clinic Foundation. "Using these products can dilate the blood vessels in your face," she says. "Over time, these vessels will stay dilated, causing reddened, irritated, blotchy skin."

Nourish skin with moisture. Skin produces less oil as we get older. How much oil it produces varies from person to person. Since oil keeps skin soft and supple, locking in your skin's moisture may be your biggest skin-care challenge.

Albert M. Kligman, M.D., Ph.D., recommends using a light, water-based moisturizer for daytime under makeup (you may try Oil of Olay Daily UV Protectant Beauty Fluid SPF 15) and a heavier, oil-based product like Nivea, Eucerin, Moisturel or even plain petroleum jelly before bed.

Makeup Tips for a Dewier, Rosier Complexion

Oil-based foundations, moisturizing powders and creamy blushers can make skin look dewier and give your complexion extra moisture. To find makeup formulated for mature skin, look for the words *hydrating, dewy* or *revitalizing* on the product's label.

"I recommend a mineral oil–based foundation for women under 50, and any creamy foundation for women 50 and up," says Marianne O'Donoghue, M.D., associate professor of dermatology at Rush Presbyterian–St. Luke's Medical Center in Chicago. But the fitter your body, the fitter your skin, says Dr. O'Donoghue. "Exercise keeps the skin in better shape," she says. "If you're really working out and perspiring profusely, you're actually cleansing your skin from the inside out. So if you're a 65-year-old-woman who plays tennis four times a week, you can use the foundation that a 35-year-old uses." But avoid oil-free foundations, oil-blotting powders and powdered blushers, which can draw attention to fine lines.

If you wear little or no makeup, reconsider. Even a hint of color on your cheeks or lips can perk up a sallow complexion. "Mature skin tends to yellow with or without sun damage," says Dr. Bergfeld. "Wearing brighter makeup can give mature skin a more youthful appearance."

The key to brightening up your face without creating an unnatural or overly made-up look is to select foundation, powder and blusher for your individual skin tone and go for subtlety. For example, mature skin is flattered by muted shades of eye shadow (say, a green shadow with a touch of brown, rather than a bright green) and cream-based lipstick in clear, strong colors like pink and coral, says Laura Geller, makeup artist and owner of Laura Geller Make-Up Studios, a cosmetics store in New York City. But avoid matte (nonshiny) lipsticks, which can make your skin look dry, and frosted eye shadows, which can give your lids a crepelike look.

Sunscreen: Young Skin in a Bottle

If you spend any amount of time outdoors during the day, you'll be pleased to learn that a $5 bottle of sunscreen or sunblock does more to make your skin look and feel younger than the most expensive moisturizer or wrinkle cream. And shielding your skin from solar assault has never been easier: You'll find lots of moisturizers and foundations formulated with added sunscreens, so you can apply sun protection along with your morning makeup.

Make sure your sunscreen has a sun protection factor (SPF) of 15 or higher, and slather it on every exposed inch of skin year-round. You may opt for a sunblock, which filters out all of the sun's punishing rays, when you'll be spending a long time in direct sunlight—on the tennis courts or the golf links, for example.

To further shield your skin, wear sunglasses to help prevent squint lines as well as cataracts, a broad-brimmed hat to further shield your face and a lip balm with added sunscreen. Your lower lip is especially vulnerable to sunburn and the unsightly changes that go with ultraviolet rays.

The Best Prescription for Lines and Crinkles

If you want more youthful-looking skin but not cosmetic surgery, ask your dermatologist about Retin-A. This cream-based derivative of vitamin A sloughs off dead cells on the surface of your skin and increases cell turnover, revealing the new skin beneath. Retin-A also stimulates the production of collagen, the material that gives skin its youthful firmness, and brightens a sallow complexion by increasing blood flow to the skin.

Generally speaking, doctors who prescribe Retin-A instruct women to apply it nightly for six months or more, then cut to about twice a week to maintain the cream's benefits. Many women start seeing results in as little as a month.

Retin-A isn't without side effects, however. After all, it is a drug. Your skin may sting, redden and burn until it gets used to the drug. A good moisturizer usually remedies these side effects. Retin-A also makes your skin exquisitely sensitive to sunlight, so during treatment you'll need to use a sunscreen with an SPF of at least 15 every time you go outdoors.

Is Cosmetic Surgery Right for You?

Cosmetic surgery can take years off your appearance, boosting your self-confidence in the bargain. But a more youthful face can't make you happier, save a relationship or change your life. So before you even schedule an appointment with a dermatologist or plastic surgeon, examine your reasons for wanting the surgery and make sure your expectations are realistic. After all, you're talking about a serious—and expensive—medical procedure.

You should also make sure you know about all the available options—surgical and nonsurgical—and what they can or cannot do. Collagen injections, facial peels and dermabrasion eliminate wrinkles but won't tighten loose, sagging skin like an eye-lift or face-lift will. All cosmetic surgery carries risks, which you should discuss with your dermatologist or surgeon at your consultation.

Do's and Don'ts for Mature Skin

Do . . .

→ Re-evaluate your skin type as you get older: You may need to switch from a routine for oily skin to a dry-skin plan.

→ Wash your face with a mild, soap-free cleansing bar, liquid cleanser or tissue-off cleansing cream formulated for dry skin.

→ Use a light, water-based moisturizer under makeup and a thicker, oil-based product at night.

→ Select a creamy foundation to give your skin a dewy appearance and perk up sallow skin with brighter shades of makeup.

→ Wear a sunscreen with an SPF of 15 year-round, and a physical sunblock when in prolonged sunlight.

→ Find out whether Retin-A may be right for you as a nonsurgical way to help acquire younger-looking skin.

Don't . . .

→ Exfoliate with abrasive pads or grainy scrubs. These products can be especially damaging to older skin.

→ Wear powdered blushers, matte lipsticks or frosted eye shadows, which don't flatter older skin.

→ Venture outdoors without sunscreen if you're using Retin-A.

→ Confuse cosmetic procedures that tighten loose, sagging skin with those that remove wrinkles.

→ Rush into cosmetic surgery without first examining your motives and expectations.

See also the chapters on puffy eyes and dark circles (chapter 14), wrinkles (chapter 20), cleansers (chapter 22), eye makeup (chapter 24), foundation, blusher and powder (chapter 25), lipstick (chapter 26), moisturizers (chapter 27), sunscreen (chapter 28) and wrinkle creams (chapter 29) and part four for more on cosmetic surgery procedures to eliminate signs of facial aging.

CHAPTER FORTY-ONE

Sun-Damaged Skin

Safeguard Your Complexion—
Whatever Your Skin Type

*D*id you get at least one bad sunburn as a child? Were you a sun worshiper as a teenager or young adult, often baking in the sun bathed in a generous coating of baby oil? Do you regularly play tennis or golf, sail, garden or power-walk in the park without first slathering on a strong sunscreen?

If you answered yes to one or more of these questions, it's likely that your skin has suffered some degree of sun damage (called photoaging)—even if you don't see it yet. That's because sun damage sneaks up on you like a thief, eventually robbing unprotected skin of its youthful appearance and turning it leathery, yellowed, blotchy and wrinkled.

Happily, it's never too late to start protecting your skin from the sun or repair even decades of sun damage. And since photoaging is every woman's concern, it's wise to add some elements of this sun-damage home-repair kit to your primary skin-care routine, regardless of your complexion, skin type or age.

Avoiding the sun and using a strong sunscreen every day are the cornerstones of this at-home program. But a dermatologist can offer further treatment options if you need them, or even help you prevent sun damage before it shows up on your skin, says Albert M. Kligman, M.D., Ph.D.

"A woman in her forties should be evaluated for underlying sun damage, even if her skin looks fine," says Dr. Kligman. "Once you're on a sun protection program, you can not only stop the damage but start to reverse it."

Even Stolen Moments in the Sun Hurt Your Skin

The majority of sun damage occurs before your 18th birthday, according to Paula A. Moynahan, M.D., attending plastic and reconstructive surgeon at Lenox Hill Hospital in New York City and St. Mary's Hospital and Waterbury Hospital in Waterbury, Connecticut. "Sun damage occurs within the skin very early in life," agrees Dr. Kligman. "But you may not see it in the mirror for decades."

What's more, it doesn't take much sun to harm your skin. "Even two bad sunburns can start the ball rolling," says Dr. Kligman. And as appealing as it may look, a suntan is just a slower type of sun damage. "Even if you always get a glorious tan, all those golden moments will add up to prematurely aged skin," he says.

Worst of all, sun damage is cumulative: Every minute you're out in the sun without sunscreen—biking through the park, driving in your car, even walking to and from the corner store—can age your skin. So anyone who's serious about maintaining youthful-looking skin needs to stop soaking in the sun and start avoiding it. The benefits: a smoother, more lustrous complexion that outglows any suntan.

Cleansing and Hydrating Sun-Dried Skin

While sun damage can affect any skin type, "it tends to affect dry skin first," says Wilma F. Bergfeld, M.D., head of clinical research and dermatopatholgy at the Cleveland Clinic Foundation. So if your skin is dry, use a creamy, soap-free cleanser or cleansing bar and a rich, oil-based moisturizer, says Dr. Bergfeld. "Fine lines and crinkles look less noticeable on moist skin," she says.

If your skin is very dry, you may try an over-the-counter alpha hydroxy acid (AHA) product like Alpha Hydrox Lotion or Avon's Anew. AHAs—mild acids derived from certain fruits, milk and sugar cane—slough away dull, dead skin cells and expose the fresh skin beneath. Many women say that using moisturizers formulated with AHAs like glycolic or lactic acid seem to brighten their skin or ease fine lines. But bear in mind that the strongest AHAs are available only from a dermatologist.

A Sure Way to Age-Proof Your Skin

The importance of using a strong sunscreen to keep your skin smoother and more youthful-looking can't be overstated: "To protect your skin, you need to use a sunscreen or sunblock every day for the rest of your life," says Dr. Moynahan.

Sunscreen and sunblock help shield your skin from the sun's most damaging rays, ultraviolet-B (UVB) and ultraviolet-A (UVA), both of which can lead to sunburns and skin cancer. UVB is primarily responsible for sunburns and skin cancer, while UVA primarily causes photoaging.

Most sunscreens generally filter UVB and some UVA. Sunblocks protect against UVA and UVB. So choose either a sunblock or a full-spectrum chemical sunscreen with a sun protection factor (SPF) of at least 15. A full-spectrum sunscreen protects against both UVA and UVB rays. Use either product every day, summer and winter. If you're fair-skinned or will be spending the day in strong sunlight—

Basic, Five-Minute Sun Protection

If you're like many people, you know wearing sunscreen protects your skin—but you keep forgetting to use it. Or you don't want to add another step to your skin-care routine. Or you just can't give up that sun-kissed glow. No more excuses: It's easier than ever to shield your skin from sun damage or give your complexion the sun-kissed glow you crave.

Simplify your sun protection. Don't want to use sunscreen, moisturizer and foundation? Streamline your beauty routine by using a moisturizer or foundation with a sun protection factor (SPF) of 15. These products offer you a convenient way to get your daily dose of sunscreen—and you'll never forget to apply it.

Use a 'screen, fake a tan. You don't have to be a "paleface" to protect your skin: One of the many self-tanners on the market can give you the sun-bronzed look you crave. But self-tanners are absolutely not a substitute for sunscreen. So don't neglect to slather on the SPF 15 whenever you step outdoors.

on the golf course or playing tennis, for example—use a sunscreen or sunblock with an SPF of 30.

Also, use the product that best suits your skin type—oil-free sunscreens if you have oily skin or chemical-free sunblocks for sensitive skin, for example.

Retin-A and AHAs:
The Dynamic Duo for Sun-Scorched Skin

Dermatologists generally treat sun-damaged skin with Retin-A (topical tretinoin)—the prescription-only vitamin A cream that's the best nonsurgical wrinkle treatment available—and prescription-strength AHAs. Says Dr. Moynahan, "Using Retin-A with AHAs increases the effectiveness of each. The aim is the same—to relieve wrinkling, smooth the skin and reduce yellowing or blotching."

Dermatologists usually have people apply Retin-A every night for six months, after which the dosage is cut to about twice a week to maintain the cream's benefits. If you have sensitive skin, a one-night-off/one-night-on Retin-A regimen may be what's called for. (You'd use a glycolic acid product on your night off.) For people whose skin can't tolerate even the lowest strength of Retin-A, some dermatologists may prescribe an AHA product only, beginning with a low (5 percent) strength and working up to a higher concentration and more frequent application.

Caution: Retin-A makes skin extremely sensitive to the sun, so you'll need to use a strong sunscreen while using this drug. To avoid future sun damage, keep slathering on the sunscreen after you stop using Retin-A.

Serious Strategies for Serious Damage

A dermatologist-administered facial peel can strip away the uppermost, superficial layer of damaged skin to reveal the newer, uncrinkled skin beneath. The strength of a facial peel can vary. A light glycolic acid peel can help eliminate slight damage, like tiny crinkles. A medium-strength trichloroacetic acid (TCA) peel can help get rid of age spots and fine lines and even out a mottled complexion. A phenol peel—the deepest peel—is reserved for only the most serious skin damage.

Don't get a stronger peel than you need, says Dr. Moynahan. "If you're in your twenties, an over-the-counter AHA product, maybe combined with a light glycolic acid peel, may be all your skin requires," she says. "If your skin is badly damaged, you may need a

TCA peel to even out blotches and eliminate some of the lines and wrinkles Retin-A leaves behind."

Many salons offer light glycolic acid peels. But a salon peel can't match the strength of a dermatologist's-office peel—generally in the 40 to 70 percent range. "A salon peel may be only 20 percent glycolic acid," notes Marianne O'Donoghue, M.D., associate professor of dermatology at Rush Presbyterian–St. Luke's Medical Center in Chicago. "While that's probably the strongest peel you should allow a salon to give you, chances are this strength won't accomplish what you want."

A further caveat: Dr. Kligman warns that some dermatologists put people on a program of peels that may be unnecessary and—worse—damaging to your skin. "Skin considers even a light peel somewhat of an insult," says Dr. Kligman. "These peels shouldn't be treated as lightly as a visit to the hairdresser."

Do's and Don'ts for Sun-Damaged Skin

Do . . .

→ Consider having a dermatologist evaluate your skin, even if you don't see evidence of sun damage.
→ Avoid the sun as much as possible.
→ Ease skin's surface dryness with a mild, soap-free cleanser and a rich moisturizer.
→ Use a full-spectrum, SPF 15 sunscreen or sunblock every day, whatever the season.
→ Use sunscreen both during and after Retin-A therapy.

Don't . . .

→ Venture outdoors without sunscreen.
→ Expect miracles from over-the-counter AHA products. The strongest AHAs are available by prescription through your dermatologist.
→ Go to a salon for a glycolic acid facial peel. Even the lightest peels should be performed in a dermatologist's office.

See also the chapters on age spots and freckles (chapter 1), sunburn (chapter 17), wrinkles (chapter 20), moisturizers (chapter 27), sunscreen (chapter 28), wrinkle creams (chapter 29), oily skin (chapter 33), dry skin (chapter 34), combination skin (chapter 35), chemical peels (chapter 45) and Retin-A (chapter 51).

CHAPTER FORTY-TWO

Acne-Prone Skin

Beautiful, Blemish-Free Skin Can Be Yours

*U*nfortunately, teenagers don't have a lock on breakouts. In fact, half of all women with adult acne escaped blemishes in their teens, says Marianne O'Donoghue, M.D., assoate professor of dermatology at Rush Presbyterian–St. Luke's Medical Center in Chicago.

Many women's late-blooming acne begins after pregnancy or during menopause, when estrogen levels soar or dip. Emotional stress can also be to blame. Fortunately, you don't have to wait to outgrow your blemishes all over again. Here's how to zap zits quick.

Cleansing Rule #1:
Try a Little Tenderness

The last thing problem skin needs is to be punished. Better to treat your troubled skin gently.

Use soaps that are easy on your skin. True soap can strip your skin and may also contain acne-triggering ingredients like sodium tallowate. So opt for a soap-free liquid soap or bar formulated for oily skin. You might use an antiseptic soap like Liquid Dial during breakouts, says Wendy E. Roberts, M.D., director of dermato-

Fewer French Fries? More Water?
Clearing Up the Two Biggest Blemish Myths

Generations of teenagers have forsworn french fries and cola in the hopes of clearing up their skin. While there are plenty of good reasons for people of all ages to avoid junk food, there's still no scientific proof that oily or sugary foods cause acne to flare. "But some people do believe that eating or drinking certain foods affects their skin," says Wendy E. Roberts, M.D., director of dermatopathology and assistant professor of dermatology at Loma Linda University Medical Center in California. And avoiding the reputed villains can't hurt. So if you think your breakouts are diet-induced, try avoiding chocolate, nuts, sugary soda, greasy foods like potato chips, and shellfish and see if you detect any improvement.

By the way, while some dermatologists believe drinking lots of water (eight glasses a day is usually the magic number) clears acne somewhat, others think chugging water merely increases your time in the bathroom.

pathology and assistant professor of dermatology at Loma Linda University Medical Center in California. But stop using an antiseptic product immediately if it irritates your skin.

Wash twice a day—no more. Despite what you may have heard, repeated cleansing won't prevent breakouts. "Too much washing can dry and irritate your skin," says Melvin L. Elson, M.D., medical director of the Dermatology Center in Nashville and co-author of *The Good Look Book*. Worse, compulsive cleansing can rile your oil glands and trigger a breakout.

Limit the astringent. Like overcleansing, using astringent more than once or twice a day can dry out—and rile up—your skin. You might try a product labeled for sensitive skin, which contains less alcohol than regular astringents.

Shun the scrubs. Because they dry up oil and temporarily tighten pores, grainy exfoliants may feel like they're helping your skin. But overusing these products can make your skin parched and flaky and can even result in tiny broken capillaries. "Trying to scrub acne away is just wrong," says Dr. Elson. Let a benzoyl peroxide product (see below) do the scrubbing for you, advises Dr. Roberts. "Its chemical exfoliation is enough."

You might also try a product formulated with salicylic acid (a chemical exfoliant thought to encourage faster cell turnover and repair), says Dr. Roberts. Neutrogena's Clear Pore Treatment, for example, is an overnight treatment that can help keep pores clear and prevent new pimples from forming.

Don't squeeze! No matter how tempted you are, never squeeze a pimple. You may push the infection deeper into your skin. Don't squeeze blackheads, either. They can be deceptively deep, and trying to extract them may break your skin, causing inflammation.

The no-squeeze rule is especially important if you're African American: Your skin may retaliate by making more pigment and replacing the pimple with a permanent dark spot.

Benzoyl Peroxide:
Your Best-Bet Zit Zapper

An over-the-counter benzoyl peroxide solution, available in 2.5, 5 and 10 percent strengths, will get rid of most run-of-the-mill pimples. For the best results, try these tips.

Use the lowest concentration. Treat mild acne with the 2.5 percent benzoyl peroxide product, says Albert M. Kligman, M.D., Ph.D. "People think the 10 percent products work better because they sting and burn, but a 2.5 percent product can be just as effective without overdrying your skin."

To help clear up a tough breakout, you might opt for a 5 percent benzoyl peroxide product. Dr. Roberts also recommends Neutrogena's Acne Mask.

Kill a blemish with kindness. Apply a benzoyl peroxide product directly on your pimples just once or twice a day—for mild acne, at night is enough—until your pimple stops being painful or itchy. "That means it's on its way out," says Wilma F. Bergfeld, M.D., head of clinical research and dermatopathology at the Cleveland Clinic Foundation. From that point on, it's hands off, she adds: A pimple takes about two weeks to heal and will fade faster if you leave it alone.

Go easy on the b.p. Overusing benzoyl peroxide can leave the skin surrounding a blemish red and flaky—not much more appealing than a blemish itself.

When Acne Flares, Don't Hide Out—Cover Up

Camouflaging blemishes can make you feel better about your skin—and in many cases, it can help clear your skin as well. You'll find plenty of medicated products that conceal while they heal and foundations that won't rile acne-prone skin.

Blemish concealers can be clear or tinted, and you can use them on bare skin or under makeup. If you prefer to use vanishing formulas, Dr. Roberts suggests Neutrogena's On-the-Spot Acne Treatment, which also absorbs excess oil. If you like tinted cover-ups, she recommends Clinique's Acne Control, which is formulated with salicylic acid.

As for foundations, Dr. Kligman recommends using products that are noncomedogenic (formulated without ingredients that are known to cause blemishes). And although you don't necessarily have to use an oil-free foundation, many women with acne-prone skin prefer oil-free or water-based makeup, which actually does contain a small amount of oil, or oil-blotting formulas that soak up shine automatically. You may want to try Clinique Stay True Oil-Free Foundation, Mary Kay Oil-Free Foundation or Ultima II Oil Control Formula Foundation. But whichever foundation you choose, "stick with well-known cosmetic brands, because they've done the most testing," advises Dr. Kligman.

Working Out without Breaking Out

Working out is good for your body. But it can be hard on your complexion: Perspiration and oil are the deadly duo of acne-prone skin. These tips can keep your skin in shape.

Wear a clean face to class. Don't wear makeup or moisturizer to the gym. "You're going to break out if you have anything on your face," says Dr. Bergfeld.

Soak up sweat. To nip blemishes in the bud, blot off perspiration midway through your workout.

Wash up after you work out. "Don't give oil a chance to block your pores while you're hanging out at the juice bar," says Dr. Berg-feld. But don't scrub, either. "Cleansing with your soap and warm or hot water will remove sweat and oil," she says.

Optional oil-blotter: astringent. While you shouldn't overuse as-tringent, it's okay to mop up postexercise oil with astringent tow-elettes. Says Dr. Roberts, "Just a few strokes of the pad across your face will refresh you." You may keep a few of these oil-busters in your workout bag.

Get out of your gear as soon as possible. Don't sit around in sweaty exercise wear, especially if it's made of spandex. Clingy fabric doesn't allow skin to breathe, which could clog pores and lead to blemishes on your back or shoulders. And always exercise in clean workout gear.

Prescription-Only Treatments for Severe Acne

If over-the-counter benzoyl peroxide products don't clear your skin in four to six weeks, consider consulting a dermatologist, ad-vises Paula A. Moynahan, M.D., attending plastic and reconstruc-tive surgeon at Lenox Hill Hospital in New York City and St. Mary's and Waterbury Hospital in Waterbury, Connecticut. "You'll be better off if you seek treatment early," she says.

Dermatologists have an arsenal of prescription-only acne treat-ments at their disposal. Two of the most effective are Retin-A (top-ical tretinoin) and Accutane (isotretinoin). Retin-A, a cream-based derivative of vitamin A that Dr. Kligman developed decades ago to treat acne, unclogs pores. Accutane, an oral drug reserved for more chronic, severe acne, virtually shuts down oil gland production, thereby shutting down blemishes. But this drug has a number of se-rious side effects. And never take Accutane if you're pregnant or think you might be; it has been linked to birth defects.

If you have mature skin, a dermatologist can devise an acne reg-imen that's right for you. "It saves time if you go right to a derma-tologist, because she knows how to handle mature skin," says Dr. O'Donoghue.

A dermatologist can also test for an underlying condition that

To Avoid Breaking Out, Try Calming Down

Some dermatologists believe stress may aggravate acne. So if you're feeling under the gun, here's how to keep stress from taking aim at your complexion.

Get moving. Beating stress can be as simple as taking a 20-minute walk or a regular yoga or meditation class. Says Wendy E. Roberts, M.D., assistant professor of dermatology at Loma Linda University Medical Center in California, "Make an hour for yourself. Bring your sneakers to work and walk during lunch. Or take an aerobics class after work."

Make a worry date with yourself. Giving yourself a set amount of time to worry—and no more—can help you deal with anxiety, says Dr. Roberts. "I often advise people to tell themselves, 'I'm going to worry on Monday from seven to eight' and then to really spend that time worrying. And then stop worrying."

could be triggering your blemishes. Small but significant fluctuations in hormone output can trigger acne in some cases. So women who have chronic acne that doesn't clear up after a variety of treatments may need a hormone level test, says Dr. Bergfeld. Estrogen or other drugs may be needed to correct the problem.

Do's and Don'ts for Acne-Prone Skin

Do . . .

→ Use a mild soap-free cleanser, never soap, to cleanse your skin.
→ Clear mild blemishes with a 2.5 percent over-the-counter benzoyl peroxide product.
→ Camouflage blemishes with tinted, medicated concealers and stick to oil-free, oil-blotting or water-based foundations.
→ Wash away perspiration and oils after you work out.
→ See a dermatologist if acne is severe.

Don't . . .

⇢ Try to scrub away pimples; it can lead to more breakouts.

⇢ Use astringent more than once or twice a day.

⇢ Use a moisturizer unless you've dried out your skin with harsh cleansing or astringents. In that case, cut back on alcohol-based products.

⇢ Squeeze blackheads or blemishes. You may aggravate them and damage your skin in the bargain.

See also the chapters on blemishes (chapter 2), cleansers (chapter 22), foundation, blusher and powder (chapter 25), moisturizers (chapter 27) and oily skin (chapter 33).

CHAPTER FORTY-THREE

Allergic Skin

Healing Hints for a Delicate Complexion

*I*f your skin often breaks into a red, itchy, bumpy rash after you use a new cleanser, moisturizer or cleanser, you most likely have allergic skin. But don't fret: Caring for this skin type doesn't necessarily have to be difficult, once you find out what you're allergic to. And while identifying the culprit or culprits can be a challenge, it's by no means impossible—and neither is keeping allergic skin smooth, clear and beautiful.

It's also a good possibility that your skin is not truly allergic but simply sensitive. (More about that in a minute.) But if you have bona fide allergic skin, your skin-care routine centers on avoiding products formulated with ingredients that rile your skin, thereby avoiding potential problems in the first place. Here's how.

Are You Really Allergic—Or Simply Sensitive?

If you think you have allergic skin, you're not alone. A survey by the American Academy of Dermatology found that 26 percent believe they have allergic skin. But you may also be mistaken: Studies estimate that allergic contact dermatitis (the medical term for a red, itchy skin rash triggered by your body's immune system) affects only 2 percent of the population.

So what's the difference between allergy and sensitivity? Alexander A. Fisher, M.D., clinical professor of dermatology at the New York University Medical Center in New York City and a specialist in allergic skin, explains: "An allergy causes the skin to change in some way—to break out in a rash or to blister—as certain cells react to the chemical or cosmetic." By contrast, a sensitivity irritation is usually invisible. Your skin is most likely sensitive if it stings for no visible reason rather than breaking out in an all-too-noticeable rash, says Dr. Fisher. More people are sensitive rather than allergic.

If you have allergic skin, you may break out in a nasty crop of hives instead of a rash. But whatever form an allergic reaction takes, don't automatically assume a skin-care product is to blame.

One woman struggled with a stubborn case of dry, flaky, itchy, red, puffy eyes—classic symptoms of eyelid dermatitis which left her miserable. Making matters worse, they left the skin around her eyes wrinkly, adding years to her face. The problem improved on weekends, when she went without makeup. After experimenting with different eye makeups, she sought the advice of a dermatologist.

As it turned out, the problem was an allergy—but not to makeup (much to her relief). The culprit was formaldehyde, commonly occurring in memos, newspapers and other paperwork the woman handled. Her hands didn't break out, but when she touched her eyes—voilà. The sensitive skin in the eye area swelled and itched. The happy ending: As long as she washes her hands before she touches her eyes, her eyelids no longer itch, swell or wrinkle.

The Four Most Common Problem Ingredients

Nevertheless, if you have allergic skin, scrutinizing skin-care products is a logical first step. Read the labels on every cleanser, moisturizer, sunscreen or cosmetic you use to check for ingredients that may rile your skin. The following ingredients are known offenders.

Fragrances. If you have allergic skin, use only products labeled fragrance-free or unscented. But despite the labeling, truly fragrance-free products are rare, says Dr. Fisher. "*Unscented* may mean only that the product has no discernible scent," he says. "The cosmetic company may have added what's called a masking fragrance to cover the odor of the product's raw ingredients."

Bear in mind that fragrance shows up in more than cleanser, moisturizer or makeup: Cinnamic alcohol and cinnamic aldehyde, for example, are in toothpaste and deodorant sanitary napkins.

Preservatives. Cosmetics companies use preservatives in skin-care products to keep them from turning rancid and causing infections, says Wilma F. Bergfeld. M.D., head of clinical research and dermatopathology at the Cleveland Clinic Foundation. But some may cause an allergic reaction: Quaternium-15, imidazolidinyl urea and parabens (methyl butyl and propyl paraben) are common offenders.

Fortunately, says Dr. Bergfeld, many cosmetics companies now use lower concentrations of several preservatives rather than a high level of just one preservative. "At a low level, a preservative is less likely to cause a reaction," she says.

Nail polish ingredients. Formaldehyde (in some nail hardeners) and toluenesulfonamide/formaldehyde resin (found in nail enamel) are common allergens. The reaction usually pops up around the neck and eyelids rather than around the nails, says Dr. Fisher, and is caused by touching your damp nails to your face or eyes. A reaction occurs only when polish is wet. So let your nails dry thoroughly before you scratch your nose or rub your eyes.

Propylene glycol. This skin softener appears in various kinds of skin-care products, from cleansers to moisturizers.

A Simple Self-Test for Allergies

A dermatologist can give you a patch test (see below), which may ferret out the ingredient or ingredients responsible for riling your skin. But unless your reaction is severe—tenderness, redness and swelling—you may try this simple use test at home before you spend valuable time and money on an office visit, says Dr. Fisher.

To do the test, dab the inside of your forearm with every one of the skin-care products you suspect of causing a reaction two or three times a day for at least four or five days, says Dr. Fisher. (Be sure to put each product on the same spot each time, so you'll know which is which.) If you're allergic to any one of them, your skin will redden and itch.

Daily Care for Allergy-Prone Skin

If you have allergic skin, use only hypoallergenic products: They generally contain fewer ingredients than regular products and few or none of the ingredients known to trigger allergic reactions.

But using only hypoallergenic products isn't a 100 percent guaranteed, fail-safe tactic. "Hypoallergenic doesn't mean *non*allergic," says

Dr. Fisher. "It just means the product is less likely to affect you. If a hypoallergenic product contains the ingredient you happen to be allergic to, it's not going to be hypoallergenic for you." Along with using hypoallergenic products, trying these tips may help save your skin.

Use the gentlest cleansers. If you can't find even a hypoallergenic cleanser your skin can tolerate, try removing your makeup with petroleum jelly. "While it's rather greasy, nobody seems to be allergic to it," says Dr. Fisher. You may also try Cetaphil, a soap-free cleanser that's known for its mildness, which you can use without water.

Make your own moisturizer. If just about every moisturizer seems to raise a rash, make your own: Blend one part olive oil with three parts water and apply your "moisturizer" cold, says Dr. Fisher. You can also moisturize with plain old petroleum jelly.

A sunblock for allergic skin. PABA (para-aminobenzoic acid), oxybenzates and most other chemical sunscreens will cause allergic skin to erupt. So choose a chemical-free sunblock formulated with titanium dioxide or zinc oxide instead, says Dr. Fisher.

Titanium dioxide can react with metals in your jewelry, leaving a black discoloration on your skin. "To avoid this, let the sunblock dry before you put on your jewelry," says Dr. Fisher.

Wearing perfume. While you may be allergic to certain fragrances (like musk ambrette, found in some men's colognes), "you don't have to give up perfume," says Dr. Fisher. If your skin reacts only when you dab perfume behind your ears, scent your forearms or behind your knees instead.

Still Stymied? Consult a Dermatologist

If a use test didn't uncover the source of your rash and you can't figure out what product or products are riling your skin, consult a dermatologist or allergist. She can give you a patch test, which tests for the 20 most common allergens and identifies the culprit for about 90 percent of people tested. One out of ten people will have to undergo further testing, says Dr. Fisher.

Once your dermatologist discovers which ingredient or ingredients are triggering the reaction, she will most likely give you a list of safe skin-care products and another of ingredients to avoid, along with the names of substances these no-no ingredients may react with. "For example, an ingredient in your moisturizer may cause a reaction when you take an antibiotic," says Dr. Fisher.

Cosmetic Procedures Aren't Out of the Question

If you have allergic skin, you don't necessarily have to rule out age-reversing cosmetic procedures. The glycolic acid used in a light facial peel, for example, rarely causes an allergic reaction, although some people are a little irritated by it, says Dr. Fisher.

Some procedures, including collagen injections to plump up wrinkles, require that you be tested beforehand to rule out the possibility of a reaction to foreign collagen. If this happens, your dermatologist can inject your own fat cells.

Do's and Don'ts for Allergic Skin

Do ...
→ Avoid using products that contain fragrances, preservatives, formaldehyde or propylene glycol.
→ Try diluted olive oil as a moisturizer substitute.
→ Use a chemical-free sunblock rather than a sunscreen.
→ Consider getting a patch test if a self-administered use test doesn't identify the offending product or products.
→ Read the chapter on sensitive skin if a patch test comes up negative: There are many things you can do to pamper delicate skin.

Don't ...
→ Rule out the possibility that something other than a skin-care product is raising a rash.
→ Assume hypoallergenic products won't trigger a reaction. They may still contain an ingredient or ingredients you're allergic to.
→ Take the word *unscented* at face value. Check a product's list of ingredients to see if it contains a masking fragrance.
→ Touch your face—especially your eyes—until your nail polish is thoroughly dry. The more coats of polish you apply, the more drying time your nails will require.
→ Start using a product you even suspect may rile your skin. Allergic reactions don't occur the first time you use the product, and you don't want to break into a rash a week or a month down the road.

See also the chapters on eczema (chapter 10), hives (chapter 11), and sensitive skin (chapter 15).

$\mathcal{D}$iabetic $\mathcal{S}$kin

Head-to-Toe Hints for Healthy Skin

*H*aving diabetes doesn't necessarily affect your complexion. But experts recommend you treat your skin with tender loving care. "If you have diabetes, you have to be very careful with your skin because your skin's ability to heal itself is compromised," says Albert M. Kligman, M.D., Ph.D. It's especially important to avoid rough treatment that invites infection—scrubbing with abrasive pads or grainy cleansers, for example.

In most other ways, however, your skin-care regimen isn't very different from that for any other skin type: Follow the routine and use the products that suit your skin type—dry, oily or combination. (You'll find those routines elsewhere in this part of the book.) And wear a sunscreen with a sun protection factor (SPF) of at least 15 every time you're outdoors—essential care for every woman's complexion.

Beyond these basics, your skin-care plan focuses on avoiding skin infections and keeping your hide healthy from the neck down.

Get on the Good Foot

People with diabetes often have circulatory problems, which can lead to nerve damage in the lower part of the body, particularly the feet. Because this nerve damage can lessen the sensation of pain, you may not notice a tiny scratch or nick on your foot that could cause a potentially serious infection: If left untreated, these infections can lead to the loss of toes, feet or worse.

So it's crucial to monitor the condition of your feet, says Steven K. Shama, M.D., clinical instructor in dermatology at Harvard Medical School. Here are his foot-healthy hints.

Keep your feet clean and dry. "Moisture tends to promote fungal and bacterial growth, so you want to do whatever you can to decrease foot moisture and humidity," says Dr. Shama. But don't scrub, he warns. "Foot care should be very gentle," says Dr. Shama. "When you wash your feet, don't rub or scrub them—that can break the skin, making infection more likely. And don't forget to thoroughly dry in between your toes."

Give your feet the once-over once a day. To keep your feet free of infection, "look for cuts or areas of redness once a day, using a hand mirror to examine the bottoms of your feet," advises Dr. Shama.

Wear the shoes that fit. "Shoes that are too tight decrease blood flow to your feet," says Dr. Shama. "And too-loose shoes can cause rubbing that can irritate your feet and form calluses." A comfortable, well-cushioned walking or running shoe that fits is a safe bet.

Don't self-doctor your dogs. If you have diabetes, don't attempt to diagnose or fix a foot problem yourself: You may not be able to judge whether the condition needs medical treatment. For example, thickened toenails, common in people who have diabetes, may be the natural result of poor circulation—or a fungal infection that needs a doctor's attention. Says Dr. Shama, "You really need to have your feet examined regularly by a podiatrist, dermatologist or vascular surgeon who's experienced in caring for the diabetic foot." Also, do not attempt to cut away or dissolve corns and calluses on your own.

To Avoid Infection, Practice Prevention

Generally speaking, women are more likely to develop yeast infections than men. What's more, "women with diabetes are more likely to get yeast infections than nondiabetic women," says Dr. Shama.

These infections like moist environments, so pay special attention to the skin in body folds, under your arms and breasts, between your toes and in the groin area. "Keep those areas as dry as possible with powder," says Dr. Shama. "Preventing an infection is much better than trying to cure one."

Take care when removing body hair, too. While you can use any method of hair removal you like—shaving, waxing, chemical depilatories, even electrolysis—you need to be careful, says Dr. Shama. "Diabetics may be at greater risk for infections of the hair follicle, so you should try any procedure in a small area first and wait a few days to see how your skin reacts," he says.

Treat Your Nails to a Manicure

Like the rest of your skin, your nails are vulnerable to infection if you have diabetes. That doesn't mean you can't indulge in a salon manicure or polish your nails yourself. But limit your manicure to shaping your nails and applying polish; don't push or snip cuticles. They're particularly vulnerable to infection. Also, be on the alert for inflammation around the cuticle or separation of the nail from the nail bed, advises Dr. Shama.

If you wear nail wraps or extensions, remove them more regularly than usual to make sure your own nails are healthy, says Dr. Shama. But if you experience tenderness around or beneath your nails, have a professional remove them at once. "Tenderness doesn't necessarily mean you have an infection," says Dr. Shama. "You may just be allergic to the glue that was placed on the nail. But no matter what the cause, it's best to seek a doctor's care."

Pay attention to the color of your nails, too. Healthy nails are pink. If yours are white or greenish-yellow, you may have a yeast or bacterial infection. "These infections sometimes occur when your blood sugar's too high," says Dr. Shama, "but they're almost always caused by doing something to your nails."

Rejuvenating Your Skin—Safely

If you have diabetes, you can renew your skin with any cosmetic procedure from dermabrasion to a face-lift, says Dr. Shama. But it's crucial that you have any procedure performed by a doctor experienced in performing the procedure on people with diabetes. And inform her of your condition: She must also monitor your condition to ensure you heal thoroughly with no harmful consequences.

"Because of the risk of infection, any kind of cosmetic procedure should be done under a doctor's supervision," says Dr. Shama. So have even a very light glycolic acid peel performed in a medical setting rather than a salon.

Do's and Don'ts for Diabetic Skin

Do...

→ Follow the skin-care regimen that suits your skin type—oily, dry or combination.

→ Inspect your feet daily, keep them clean and dry and wear comfortable footwear to sidestep potentially serious foot infections.

→ Powder your skin to keep it dry, especially in between body folds: Trapped moisture breeds infection-causing bacteria.

→ Try any hair-removal method, including shaving, waxing, chemical depilatories and electrolysis on a small area of skin before attempting a larger area.

→ Limit both professional and self-manicures to shaping and polishing only.

→ Remove nail wraps or artificial nails more regularly than usual to make sure your nails are healthy.

→ Pursue cosmetic surgery, but have a doctor monitor your recovery for any sign of infection.

Don't...

→ Overwash your face or use abrasive products that could break the skin.

→ Forget to wear sunscreen with an SPF of at least 15.

→ Self-treat any foot condition, including corns and calluses. Consult a podiatrist or other specialist who's experienced in treating the feet of people with diabetes.

→ Self-diagnose or self-treat skin problems, especially on the feet. Consult your doctor instead.

→ Let a manicurist cut or trim your cuticles or cut or trim them yourself.

→ Go to a salon for even a light facial peel.

See also the chapters on blisters, calluses and corns (chapter 3), sunscreen (chapter 28), oily skin (chapter 33), dry skin (chapter 34), combination skin (chapter 35), chemical peels (chapter 45), cosmetic surgery (chapter 47) and dermabrasion (chapter 48).

PART FIVE

Medical Options for Age Reversal

CHAPTER FORTY-FIVE

Chemical Peels

Unveil a Fresher, Smoother Complexion

Throughout this book, one message comes through loud and clear: If you want more beautiful, youthful-looking skin, slather on the sunscreen. The good news is, every drop of sunscreen you use now can prevent sun damage in the future. But if years of baking on the beach, lying in tanning beds or engaging in outdoor sports without sun protection has left your skin less smooth and radiant than it could be, you may be a good candidate for a facial peel. This nonsurgical procedure can help eliminate some or virtually all of the youth-robbing effects of sun damage, including wrinkling. There's also some evidence that facial peels may help the skin to generate collagen, the substance that helps the skin stay firm and taut.

In a facial peel, a dermatologist applies one of several chemical acids to the face and peels away the upper layers of dull, damaged skin. "A facial peel is a chemical burn that induces healing—old skin peels off and new skin replaces it," says Melvin L. Elson, M.D., medical director of the Dermatology Center in Nashville and co-author of *The Good Look Book*.

If undergoing a facial peel sounds drastic, it is: This procedure isn't risk-free, and it isn't right for everyone. But for certain people, and when performed by a qualified doctor, a facial peel can deliver more youthful-looking skin.

The Appeal of Peels

There are three basic types of peels: light, medium and deep. A light peel freshens skin by removing only the top layer of skin. A medium peel penetrates more deeply into the skin and can help eliminate fine wrinkles and blotches. A deep peel can help eliminate deeper wrinkles, benign skin growths and more severe sun damage.

Which type of peel is best for you depends on how much sun damage your skin has sustained. "Light peels can freshen the skin and make it look a little smoother and prettier, while medium or deep peels can eliminate some wrinkling," says Dr. Elson. The color of your skin may also be a factor (see below).

Many dermatologists have people pretreat their skin with Retin-A (topical tretinoin), the prescription vitamin A cream used to fight wrinkles, for up to a month before a peel. "Retin-A increases the fibro-

Should You Get a Salon Peel?

Walk into any salon or day spa, and chances are you'll be able to get a light peel. But undergoing even a superficial peel in a salon rather than in a dermatologist's office can be ineffective at best and dangerous at worst, say experts.

A salon peel may be too light to be of benefit, says Melvin L. Elson, M.D., medical director of the Dermatology Center in Nashville and co-author of *The Good Look Book*. "You may end up losing dollars, not wrinkles." Adds Albert M. Kligman, M.D., Ph.D., "If you're looking for serious results, have even a light peel performed by a qualified dermatologist."

There's also the risk that light salon peels aren't as light as you think. Many states don't regulate peels, notes Steven J. Pearlman, M.D., facial plastic surgeon and president of the New York Facial Plastic Surgery Society in New York City. "Some salons may be giving very strong peels, and using the higher percentages of glycolic acid is potentially dangerous," he says. Any peel other than a very mild glycolic acid peel should be performed under a doctor's supervision, he says. Dr. Elson goes even further: "Because of the potential risks, salon peels should be removed from the market."

blasts—the cells that make collagen—and increases the blood flow in the skin," explains Dr. Elson. And a month before a medium or deep peel, a doctor may do a patch test at your hairline to see how your skin will react to whatever acid solution will be used. But a patch test can't predict how skin will react to a full-face chemical peel, says Dr. Elson.

Unhappily, facial peels—especially medium and deep peels—can be painful. A dermatologist usually administers a combination of drugs, often intravenously, to help ease the pain.

Your doctor will fill you in on how to care for your skin after a peel. But generally speaking, postpeel skin care entails gentle cleansing, frequent moisturizing and staying out of the sun (see below for more on the importance of sun protection).

Tired-Looking Skin? Perhaps a Light Peel Will Do

If your skin doesn't look as smooth or fresh as it used to, you may opt for a light peel, which removes dead cells on the surface of your skin. Many dermatologists perform light peels with glycolic acid, one of the alpha hydroxy acids (AHAs)—mild acids derived from natural substances like fruit, milk and sugar cane. The glycolic acid used in a light peel is the same stuff cosmetics companies put in their moisturizers, only stronger.

Generally speaking, the glycolic acid is left on the skin for up to seven minutes, then washed off with water. Your skin may sting during the procedure, and afterward you'll probably look like you have a mild sunburn.

Some experts say that undergoing regular glycolic acid peels can help improve the quality of your skin faster than using a glycolic acid moisturizer alone. But not all dermatologists think that perpetual peels are good for skin. "In places like Miami and Hollywood, some dermatologists give people glycolic acid peels every two to three weeks," says Albert M. Kligman, M.D., Ph.D. "A lot of women are on a schedule—it's like going to the hairdresser. But without some serious study, it's risky to undergo these peels for a long period of time."

Lift Away Even More Damage

If your skin has more than superficial sun damage, your doctor may suggest a medium peel. Most dermatologists use trichloroacetic acid (TCA), which is formulated in a variety of concentrations and matched to the depth of lines and wrinkles. TCA peels vary in strength—20 percent for a light peel to 35 to 50 percent for a medium or deep peel. Medium peels are particularly effective on fine lines around the eyes and deep lines around the mouth, says Dr. Elson.

Most doctors agree that fair-skinned people benefit most from a TCA peel, and that medium peels are riskier for people with medium or dark skin. There is the occasional exception: Harold E. Pierce, Jr., M.D., dermatologist and cosmetic surgeon at the Pierce Cosmetic Surgery Center in Philadelphia and professor emeritus of dermatologic cosmetic surgery at Howard University in Washington, D.C., says that TCA peels can also be safe for black skin (see below for more on peels and black skin).

For maximum effect, doctors will often administer a light peel, like the Jessner's peel, immediately before they perform a TCA peel. "A Jessner's peel allows a lower concentration of TCA to penetrate more deeply into the skin, which increases the benefits without increasing the risk of scarring," says Dr. Elson.

TCA peels can be painful: Expect ten minutes of severe pain, from the time the solution is applied to the time it's washed off, says Dr. Elson. The pain can last for a day or two. His advice: You can ease the discomfort by taking an over-the-counter pain reliever.

After a TCA peel, skin usually frosts, or turns white. It then turns red, scabs and peels. But most people who undergo a TCA peel can go out without makeup or with very little makeup in seven or eight days.

The Peel of All Peels

The deepest chemical peel of all is the phenol peel, in which the entire outer layer of the epidermis and part of the dermis are burned away. A phenol peel can remove severe sun damage and make deep wrinkles appear less noticeable. But the benefits of this procedure must be weighed against its risks: "A phenol peel is by far the most effective," says Dr. Kligman, "but it's also the riskiest."

A phenol peel destroys skin's melanocytes, the cells that contain pigment. So most people who undergo a phenol peel will have permanently lighter skin than before the peel. There's also a chance that skin could become completely depigmented, which is why a phenol peel works best on fair, dry, thin skin. Phenol peels aren't recommended for people with medium, dark or black skin.

Phenol peels are also extremely painful—especially afterward— and skin can remain red for three to four months. A phenol peel also makes skin more sensitive to the sun than before, so you'll need to completely avoid the sun for the first six months after the procedure and wear a strong sunscreen forever after.

Most alarmingly, however, phenol is absorbed through the skin and can cause an irregular heartbeat if it's applied too quickly. So great is this potential risk that people undergoing a phenol peel are hooked up to a cardiac monitor, and doctors apply the phenol to one area of the face at a time to avoid releasing too much phenol into the blood-stream. "The entire peel can take two or three hours," says Dr. Elson. It's also possible for phenol to damage the liver and kidneys. So *never* undergo a phenol peel if you have a heart, liver or kidney condition.

With all these risks, it's a wonder anyone undergoes a phenol peel at all. Some experts suggest that people considering a phenol peel opt for a TCA peel instead. "A high-strength TCA peel can border on the strength of a phenol peel without causing the serious health risks," says William B. Rosenblatt, M.D., attending plastic surgeon at Lenox Hill Hospital in New York City.

To Peel or Not to Peel

Before signing up for any chemical peel, you should know about the risks. The deeper the peel, the higher the risk. You should discuss these potential complications with the doctor before you schedule an appointment for any type of peel, and make sure you understand and are satisfied with his or her answers to your questions.

Possible complications include temporary and permanent changes in the color of the skin. If you're African American, you should know that getting a medium or deep peel puts you at risk of losing some portion of your skin color. Scarring—the result of burning too deeply into the skin and triggering an abnormal collagen growth—is also a possibility.

In rare cases, getting a facial peel can reactivate the herpes simplex virus in susceptible people or cause an infection that will need to be treated with drugs.

Also, know what a facial peel can't do. "A peel can't eliminate deep furrows, not even a phenol peel," says Steven J. Pearlman, M.D., facial plastic surgeon and president of the New York Facial Plastic Surgery Society in New York City. Nor can facial peels fix deep folds: The only remedy for sagging skin is cosmetic surgery.

See also the chapter on cosmetic surgery (chapter 47).

CHAPTER FORTY-SIX

Collagen Injections and Other Filler Techniques

Look Years Younger in Days

$\mathcal{B}$othered by crow's-feet that linger, no matter how much sunscreen and moisturizer you slather on? Annoyed by tiny whistle lines around your mouth, or forehead furrows that leave you looking older than your years? Or tiny scars on an otherwise well-maintained complexion? Don't fret: A dermatologist or cosmetic surgeon can temporarily plump up fine lines, wrinkles and acne scars by injecting them with collagen and other substances.

Filler techniques are quick and relatively painless. Best of all, they can help make your skin look fresher and more youthful—without surgery. "Filler substances can reverse some of the signs of aging and sun damage," says Kevin S. Pinski, M.D., dermatologist, cosmetic surgeon and assistant professor at Northwestern University Medical Center in Chicago.

Here's the catch: The benefits of filler substances generally last less than a year—sometimes less than six months. Further, filler procedures entail a small amount of risk. But if you don't mind the maintenance this procedure requires, or you just want to avoid the long healing period and the more serious complications associated with some other cosmetic procedures, you may want to explore filler techniques. Here's what you need to know.

Rout Wrinkles with Collagen

To plump up wrinkles, most dermatologists and cosmetic surgeons use bovine collagen, which is processed from cowhide and is similar to the collagen in our own skin. "Collagen injections can make expression lines appear softer," says Melvin L. Elson, M.D., medical director of the Dermatology Center in Nashville and co-author of *The Good Look Book*.

Collagen injections work best on crow's-feet, lines around the lips, the fold that extends from each side of the nose to the corners of the mouth (called the nasolabial line) and furrows between the eyebrows. Doctors use one of two collagen formulas: Zyderm for fine lines, like those around the eyes, and Zyplast for deeper lines. Both formulas contain 3½ percent collagen and over 90 percent water.

Before the injections, a doctor may give you two patch tests to rule out an allergy to collagen. She may also have you use Retin-A (topical tretinoin)—the prescription-only vitamin A cream used to treat both wrinkles and acne—for up to a month before the injections. Retin-A increases the skin's supply of fibroblasts, the cells that make collagen, explains Dr. Elson. "If the fibroblasts are already making collagen in the area to be injected, the injected collagen will work better and last longer," he explains.

The collagen itself is injected into the lines or wrinkles with extremely fine needles. A doctor can do a lip augmentation (in which thinning lips are plumped with collagen) in about 5 minutes, eliminate crow's-feet in about 30 minutes and treat an assortment of wrinkles on the forehead, around the eyes and around the mouth in about an hour. Collagen injections can also soften shallow, saucer-shaped acne scars.

Collagen injections can be somewhat painful, says Dr. Elson. The collagen solution contains a small amount of a local anesthetic, however, which helps numb the area.

Afterward, the injected skin may bruise. But most often, the area will experience some puffiness that fades in minutes. "You can usually apply makeup and leave right after the procedure," says Dr. Elson.

The down side of collagen injections is that they usually don't last very long. "While acne scars treated with collagen may last three or four years, a lip augmentation lasts six weeks," says Dr. Elson. So for the benefits to last, you'll need additional injections.

You may have to touch up "active" parts of your face—like the nasolabial line and lines around the lips and mouth—every four to six months, says Dr. Elson. On the other hand, crow's-feet injected with collagen may stay plumped for as long as a year. And furrows between the eyebrows may stay smooth for at least nine months, says Dr. Elson.

How durable collagen injections can be also depends on a doctor's skill, says Dr. Elson. Inexperienced doctors may not inject enough collagen or may not inject it deeply enough. Says Dr. Elson, "A doctor who performs one injection every few weeks can't give you the same results as a doctor who performs one injection an hour."

De-age Skin with a Fat Transplant

Hard to believe, but doctors can use your own body fat to plump up wrinkles. In so-called autologous fat transplant procedures a cosmetic surgeon draws fat or collagen from one part of your body (usually the thigh) with a syringe or a small instrument called a cannula and reinjects this material into the layer of fat just under the skin. You'll be given local anesthesia, so the procedure isn't generally painful. You may experience minor bruising, swelling and redness, however, which usually last for a day.

Dr. Pinski prefers to use autologous body fat or collagen rather than bovine collagen to fix age-related fat loss in the face and deep expression lines. While autologous fat by itself is too thick to treat fine lines and wrinkles, a doctor can turn it into a finer, gel-like substance used to fill fine lines.

Autologous collagen lasts about as long as bovine collagen. Autologous fat may last longer, however. "After three months, only a third of the initial fat injections may remain," says Dr. Pinski. "But with touch-ups, you may be able to get some permanent results."

Dermal Grafts: They Last and Last . . .

Strictly speaking, a dermal graft isn't a filler treatment. But it performs like one: In this procedure, a cosmetic surgeon uses a small piece of skin from behind the ear or around the groin to soften deep nasolabial folds, minimize frown lines between the eyebrows and plump up thinning lips. "Dermal grafts are permanent, or nearly permanent," says James W. Smith, M.D., associate attending surgeon at New York Hospital–Cornell Medical Center in New York City.

Dermal grafts are performed under local anesthesia, so there's little pain, if any. And there's virtually no visible scarring because all the incisions are hidden in natural creases in the skin. Dermal grafts don't work on tiny wrinkles like crow's-feet, however.

What to Know before You Go

Collagen injections and other injectable fillers can't fix sun-induced pigment changes like roughness, blotchiness or sagging skin. And while collagen works especially well on crow's-feet and the nasolabial line, it's less effective for whistle lines around the mouth, says Dr. Pinski.

"Most of the time, collagen injections are very safe," says Dr. Pinski. But they're not risk-free. Side effects—for example, an abscess or ulceration—are rare but serious and may take months to heal or cause permanent scarring.

There's also been some evidence that in some people, collagen injections can trigger an autoimmune disorder called polymyositis/dermatomyositis (PM/DM), a progressive weakening of the muscles. But this hasn't yet been proven conclusively.

Fibrel: Falling Out of Favor?

When Fibrel, a filler substance derived from pig hides, was first introduced, it seemed like a viable alternative for people allergic to bovine collagen. Fibrel was also supposed to last longer than collagen—up to five years. But some experts say Fibrel hasn't performed as well as doctors had originally hoped. "In general, it's the least effective of the fillers," says Albert M. Kligman, M.D., Ph.D.

Because it's not as thin as collagen, Fibrel can't be used to treat fine lines. Also, this substance has to be mixed with your own blood—time-consuming for the doctor and somewhat uncomfortable for you.

Worse, Fibrel tends to cause more side effects than bovine collagen. "Fibrel causes a great deal of pain and a lot of bruising," says Dr. Elson. In some people, inflammation can last up to six weeks. As for Fibrel's staying power? Says Dr. Elson, "When I used it, its effects were gone in a couple of weeks."

Dr. Pinski says that, in his experience, Fibrel doesn't have anything collagen doesn't. "If someone is allergic to bovine collagen, I would generally use autologous collagen," he says.

CHAPTER FORTY-SEVEN

Cosmetic Surgery

Is It Right for You?

*E*ver considered getting a face-lift to erase the sags and bags that make you look older than you feel? You're not alone. But if you dropped the idea because the word *face-lift* made you think of an aging movie queen whose "fixed" face looks more like a porcelain mask than flesh and blood, you have a lot to learn about cosmetic surgery.

Performed correctly, today's cosmetic procedures—which include the face-lift as well as "spot treatments" that can de-age the eyes, nose, neck and forehead—are subtle and natural-looking. In other words, cosmetic surgery can make you look like a younger version of *you*, not an expressionless department-store mannequin.

And cosmetic surgery isn't just for celebrities anymore. "Fifty years ago, only movie stars or eccentrics had face-lifts. But that's changed," says cosmetic surgeon Marjorie Cramer, M.D., clinical assistant professor of surgery at St. Vincent's Hospital and Medical Center in New York City and founder and owner of the Cramer Center for Cosmetic Surgery. In 1992, almost a half-million Americans gathered their courage (and perhaps maxed out their credit cards) and sought a surgical solution to the inexorable march of time. What's more, it seems, you're never too old for cosmetic surgery: While most women who underwent a cosmetic procedure in 1992 were ages 35 to 50, almost 30 percent were age 50 and over.

But there's more to cosmetic surgery than smoothing sags and wrinkles. Done for the right reasons, cosmetic surgery can give a person what might be called an emotional makeover as well as a physical one.

Done for the *wrong* reasons, however, getting a face-lift can be a real letdown. "Unlike in the movies, cosmetic surgery doesn't change the face drastically," says Steven J. Pearlman, M.D., facial plastic surgeon and president of the New York Facial Plastic Surgery Society in New York City. Nor can cosmetic surgery make you look like a kid again. "I think of a face-lift as a way to turn back the clock a few years," says Dr. Cramer. "But that clock keeps ticking."

And while getting an eye tuck might not be nearly as serious as undergoing heart surgery, make no mistake—cosmetic surgery isn't risk-free. Nor are its benefits instantaneous: You won't look young and beautiful the moment the bandages come off. (In fact, you may look downright horrendous.)

In short, cosmetic surgery is serious business. So before you decide to take the plunge, you owe it to yourself to investigate the alternatives to surgery (see "At a Glance: Common Medical Options for Age Reversal" on page 262). But if you feel that artfully applied makeup and a flattering hairstyle can no longer hide the passing of the years or that other medical treatments can't address your needs, cosmetic surgery may be an option. Here's what you need to know to make an informed decision.

One from Column A . . .

Surprise: You may not need a face-lift at all. One or more of these surgical "spot treatments" can help take years off your appearance.

Even better, cosmetic surgeons can perform these and most other cosmetic procedures in their offices or other nonhospital setting. So in most cases, people can go home the day of surgery.

Brow-lift: This procedure tightens the forehead and brow area, lifts droopy upper eyelids and softens furrows across the forehead and between the eyebrows.

To perform a brow-lift, a surgeon makes an ear-to-ear incision across the scalp at or within the hairline. After suturing, the brow is automatically lifted. A brow-lift takes about an hour to perform and is usually permanent: "Few people need more than one brow-lift," says Dr. Pearlman. Most people can resume their normal routine

Shopping for a Surgeon? Give 'Em the Third Degree

A consultation is your chance to examine a surgeon's credentials—and your gut feeling about her. Here's what to ask during this important interview.

Did you train in cosmetic surgery? If you don't see medical certificates on the wall, or if a surgeon acts cagey about her medical training, "consumer beware," says William B. Rosenblatt, M.D., attending plastic surgeon at Lenox Hill Hospital in New York City.

Are you board certified? Surgeons who perform cosmetic surgery should be certified by the American Board of Plastic Surgery or by the American Board of Otolaryngology and Head and Neck Surgery.

Will you conduct the consultation yourself? In some practices, the person who does the consultation is an employee whose job is to sign you up for surgery. (This is especially true of free consultations.) "You get what you pay for, so pay for a consultation with the doctor who will perform the surgery," says Dr. Rosenblatt.

How often do you perform this type of surgery? Says Marjorie Cramer, M.D., clinical assistant professor of surgery at St. Vincent's Hospital and Medical Center in New York City and founder and owner of the Cramer Center for Cosmetic Surgery,

within a week, says William B. Rosenblatt, M.D., attending plastic surgeon at Lenox Hill Hospital in New York City. But your forehead or scalp may be numb for a couple of months "because the procedure stretches a certain nerve," says Dr. Pearlman. (These areas will tingle as sensation returns.)

If you just want to get rid of vertical lines between the eyebrows (which can sometimes make people look angry or depressed), your surgeon might suggest an endoscopic brow-lift. In this one-hour procedure, a surgeon uses an endoscope—a surgical telescope—to cut the corrugator muscle, which causes these furrows.

Be warned, however: While some surgeons say that furrows treated with an endoscope tend to stay plumped longer than lines injected with collagen, others claim that this procedure isn't as effective as a regular brow-lift.

"You don't want a surgeon whose practice is 99 percent burn patients and 1 percent face-lifts."

Do you offer computer imaging? In computer imaging, a photo of you is manipulated on a computer to show you what you'd look like after various cosmetic procedures. But if you meet with a surgeon who offers this service, "the surgeon—not a secretary or consultant—should do the imaging," says Dr. Rosenblatt.

Can I meet with one of your patients who had the surgery I'm considering? The surgeon will naturally put you in touch with someone who raves about the results of the surgery (and the surgeon). Still, you might find it helpful to get a firsthand account of the surgery from someone who's been through it. "You'll also get an idea of how concerned and available the doctor is," says Dr. Cramer.

Can I call you at any hour, if necessary, immediately after the surgery? "There's nothing worse than calling your doctor with a problem and hearing a recording that says to call back tomorrow," says Dr. Rosenblatt. "You want a doctor whose office answers the phone at midnight."

Above all, trust your instincts. Says Dr. Cramer, "If your gut feeling about one doctor is negative, arrange a consultation with another."

Eyelid surgery (blepharoplasty): One of the most requested of all spot procedures, blepharoplasty tightens sagging upper lids and removes bags under the eyes. This so-called eyelid-lift can help make you look fresher, more alert and years younger. A surgeon makes incisions in the crease of the upper lids or just below the lashline of the lower lids. She then separates skin from underlying tissue and muscle, removes excess fat and trims drooping skin and muscle. The eyelid-lift takes about 20 minutes per lid, says Dr. Pearlman, and lids can remain taut for 10 to 15 years.

If you want to get rid of fatty pouches under your eyes, a surgeon might recommend transconjunctival blepharoplasty. In this one-hour procedure, a doctor makes an incision inside the lower lid and removes fatty bags with no visible external scar.

Nasal tip plasty: Gravity and time can pull down the nose, making the tip droop toward the mouth. "Tip plasty lifts the end of the nose and eliminates this droop," says Dr. Cramer. In this hour-long procedure, a surgeon makes tiny incisions inside the nose and repositions or removes nasal cartilage to lift the tip. "Afterward, most people can return to their normal routine, except for exercise, within a week," says Dr. Pearlman. Your nose should remain uptilted for 15 to 20 years.

Cheek implants (malar augmentation): If your cheeks have lost their youthful plumpness, this procedure can help correct a gaunt, drawn look. "A surgeon can either give you higher cheekbones or fill in the area beneath the cheekbones, which becomes sunken with age," says Dr. Cramer.

A surgeon inserts cheek implants from inside your mouth, so you won't have visible scars, says Dr. Cramer. What's more, your cheeks will remain full indefinitely.

Chin implants (mentoplasty): If you want to re-form a receding chin, a surgeon can insert a chin implant from the inside of the mouth or through a small incision under the chin. Like a cheek implant, this procedure usually takes about an hour—and improvement is usually permanent.

Lip advancement: If your lips have thinned with age, this procedure can replump them in about an hour. A surgeon makes an incision along the lipline and removes a strip of skin next to it. She then stitches the remaining skin to the edge of the lipline, which creates a new lipline and fuller lips. In most cases, lips will remain permanently full, says Dr. Pearlman.

Neck-lift: This procedure can help firm up a saggy chicken neck and turkey gobbler chin. (A neck-lift can't eliminate jowls, however.) In a neck-lift, a surgeon makes small incisions just behind or around each ear, plus a third under the chin. Then she pulls up excess skin and tightens underlying muscles. Your neck and chin will most likely remain taut for 10 to 15 years.

Do the "Tighten Up"

In the early years of cosmetic surgery, surgeons performing a face-lift pulled sagging skin as tight as a hospital bedsheet, leaving the sagging muscles *under* the skin untouched. That's why many people who underwent a face-lift (technically called a rhytidectomy) looked like they'd just stepped out of a wax museum.

Now, most surgeons also lift the submuscular aponeurotic system

(SMAS)—the layer of connective tissue that encompasses the facial muscles—as well as the skin itself. The result: Today's face-lift looks subtle, natural and relaxed.

Your face is unique, so your face-lift will be, too. Generally speaking, however, a surgeon makes incisions at each temple within the hairline, which extend in front of the ear and curve behind the earlobe. She then separates skin from underlying fat and muscle, tightens the muscles, pulls back the skin and trims away the excess.

There are three basic types of face-lifts: the standard face-lift, the deep plane face-lift and the composite face-lift. In a standard face-lift, a surgeon works on the lower third of the face to eliminate jowls and trim the chin, jawline and neck. In a deep plane face-lift, which addresses the middle third of the face, a surgeon softens the line that runs from each side of the nose to the mouth (called the nasolabial fold). In a composite face-lift, a surgeon tightens the whole face. It takes three to five hours to perform a standard face-lift and up to seven hours to do a deep plane or composite face-lift.

A standard face-lift lasts five to ten years. "It may last even longer if you get it in your forties," says Dr. Rosenblatt.

What to Expect after Surgery

As mentioned, you'll most likely be able to go home the day of surgery. But you'll probably be required to have someone accompany you home. What's more, you'll most likely welcome having a friend or your spouse nearby: You may not want to tend to yourself for the first few days. "You'll want to take it easy for the first day or two after surgery," says Dr. Rosenblatt. You'll see your surgeon for a follow-up visit anywhere from a day to a week after surgery.

You may feel discomfort, or even pain, for a few days, and your doctor may prescribe a prescription pain reliever. "An over-the-counter pain reliever like Tylenol is usually enough to ease your discomfort after the first few days," says Dr. Pearlman.

You may be able to take the pain better than you will your appearance, though. Be prepared to look like a prizefighter for a few weeks at least: Bruising and swelling can be fierce and can linger from a few weeks for most spot procedures to one month for a standard face-lift. (If you opt for a deep plane or composite face-lift, says Dr. Pearlman, "You may want to hide out for more than a month.")

Postsurgery bruising and swelling can throw some people into a
(continued on page 264)

At a Glance: Common Medical Options for Age Reversal

Procedure: Retin-A
De-aging action: Stimulates production of collagen, which gives skin its youthful appearance. Encourages the growth of new blood vessels, which gives skin a youthful glow. Sloughs away dead skin cells, uncovering new skin beneath.
Recovery time: Not applicable.
Potential risks: May turn skin red, flaky and irritated. Your dermatologist may lower the strength or frequency of application.
Additional comments: Retin-A makes skin *extremely* sensitive to sunlight, so wear a strong sunscreen every time you go outdoors.
Doctors say: "The more damaged your skin, the more improvement you'll see."—Albert M. Kligman, M.D., Ph.D.

Procedure: Chemical peel
De-aging action: Light peel: "Freshens" skin. Medium peel: Can help eliminate fine wrinkles and skin coarseness. Deep peel: Can help eliminate deeper wrinkles and severe sun damage.
Recovery time: Light peel: None. (Skin may look like it has a mild sunburn.) Medium peel: Skin usually "frosts," then turns red, scabs and peels. Most people can go with no makeup (or very little) in 7 or 8 days. Deep peel: Can take up to 2 weeks to scab over and heal; skin can remain red for 3 to 4 months.
Potential risks: Light peel: No known risks. Medium and deep peels: Scarring. Milia. Hypopigmentation (light spots) or hyperpigmentation (dark spots), especially with medium or dark skin.
Additional comments: A dermatologist may give you a patch test a month before a medium or deep peel to see how your skin reacts to the chemical solution. Medium or deep peels work best on fair-skinned people and are riskier for people with medium or dark skin. Facial peels—especially medium and deep peels— can be painful. You may need to use camouflage makeup permanently to hide hypopigmentation (light spots). Phenol used in deep peels can damage heart, liver and kidneys. People who take the acne drug Accutane may be more likely to develop scars after dermabrasion.
Doctors say: "A high-strength tricholoracetic acid (medium) peel can border on the strength of a phenol (deep) peel without causing phenol's serious health risks." —William B. Rosenblatt, M.D.

Procedure: Collagen injections
De-aging action: Fills in crow's-feet, laugh lines around the lips, nose-to-mouth lines and furrows between the eyebrows.
Recovery time: Usually none; results are virtually immediate.
Potential risks: Temporary swelling and bruising. Allergic reaction to collagen. Skin abscess (rare).
Additional comments: Before the injections, a doctor may give you patch tests to rule out an allergy to collagen. Injections can be somewhat painful: Expect more discomfort around the mouth, less around the eyes. Injected area may be puffy afterward; this usually fades within minutes. Benefits are temporary; touchups are required every few months.
Doctors say: "Schedule a touch-up when you start to notice that you don't look as good as you did right after the injections." —Melvin L. Elson, M.D.

Procedure: Liposuction
De-aging action: On face: Can slim double chin, puffy neck or jowls. On body: Can remove excess fat from problem areas like the hips, thighs, abdomen and buttocks. *May* improve the appearance of cellulite.
Recovery time: Face: Bandages removed in 24 hours. A minilift will cause swelling or bruising. Body: 4 to 5 days. Swelling disappears gradually; may take 3 to 6 months to see maximum results.
Potential risks: While a newer technique has significantly reduced liposuction's potential for complications, possible risks include dimpled skin, diminished sensation in the treated area, scarring and allergic reaction to anesthesia.
Additional comments: Facial liposuction: Works best for people in their thirties or forties whose skin is resilient enough to snap back by itself. A minilift can cause facial bruising or swelling; you'll have to wear a facial support garment for a week to 10 days. Body liposuction: You'll have to wear 2 elastic support garments for 2 to 5 days. Won't eliminate cellulite but may improve its appearance.
Doctors say: "People who undergo liposuction should be within 20 percent of desirable body weight."—Dwight Scarborough, M.D.

(continued)

At a Glance—Continued

Procedure: Eye-lift
De-aging Action: Tightens droopy upper lids or baggy lower lids. May remove some wrinkles along with excess skin.
Recovery time: Bruising and swelling fades in 2 to 3 weeks.
Potential risks: Temporary swelling and bruising. Hematoma (bleeding under the skin). Temporary blurred vision. Dry eyes or excessive tearing. Scarring. Temporary difficulty closing eyes (sometimes permanent). Blindness (very rare).
Additional comments: Cold compresses can help reduce swelling immediately after surgery. You generally can't wear contact lenses for about 2 weeks; they may feel uncomfortable even then. Your eyes will be sensitive to sunlight, wind and other irritants for several weeks; wear sunglasses outdoors.
Doctors say: "Don't apply eye makeup for about 2 weeks after surgery—the skin is much too delicate."—Marjorie Cramer, M.D.

Procedure: Dermabrasion
De-aging action: Improves texture and tone of skin. Helps remove age spots and acne scars. Eradicates some wrinkles around eyes and lips and on forehead and cheeks. Softens very deep expression lines.
Recovery time: After about 1 week, dermabraded skin looks sunburned. It may take 3 months to return to normal color.
Potential risks: Swelling. Milia. Skin lightening (may be permanent). Skin darkening (can be corrected). Chance of scarring. Infection (rare).
Additional comments: Dermabrasion tends to produce better results on fair skin. You must avoid the sun for 3 months and use sunscreen forever after. If you continue bad habits (sunbathing and smoking), skin damage will recur.
Doctors say: "If you have medium or dark skin, opt for full-face dermabrasion, rather than a spot treatment, like above the upper lip."—John M. Yarborough, M.D.

funk. "Some people do feel a little depressed after surgery," says Dr. Pearlman. But depression, while rare, is normal and usually temporary, say experts.

Also, most people who undergo a cosmetic procedure can resume

Procedure: Brow-lift
De-aging action: Tightens the forehead and brow area. Lifts droopy
upper eyelids. Softens furrows across the forehead and between
the eyebrows.
Recovery time: About 1 month. Forehead or scalp may be numb for
2 months from the stretching of a nerve.
Potential risks: Hair loss along the incision. If the nerve is damaged,
forehead or scalp numbness could be permanent.
Additional comments: At this writing, some surgeons say the endoscopic brow-lift isn't as effective on vertical furrows between
the eyebrows as the standard brow-lift.
Doctors say: "If you also need an eye-lift, schedule that procedure
for 3 months after a brow-lift. If you undergo too much surgery
at one time, you may have difficulty closing your eyes."—
Steven J. Pearlman, M.D.

Procedure: Face-lift
De-aging action: Standard face-lift: Eliminates jowls; trims the chin,
jawline and neck. Deep plane face-lift: Softens the nose-to-
mouth line (nasolabial fold). Composite face-lift: Tightens the
whole face.
Recovery time: Bruising: 1 to 6 weeks. Swelling: 2 months for a standard face-lift; 3 months for a deep plane or composite face-lift.
Potential risks: Hair loss along the hairline. Temporary numbness of
the face. Hematoma. Skin slough (tissue death). Allergic reaction
to anesthesia. Scarring. Infection or nerve damage (rare).
Additional comments: Your face may appear distorted and facial
movements may be stiff for some time after surgery, and your
skin may feel rough and dry for several months. Length of
healing period and risks increase in proportion to the depth of
the lift.
Doctors say: "Depending on the swelling and bruising, you could be
back to work in a week to 10 days."—William B. Rosenblatt, M.D.

their regular routine a few days after surgery—with minor restric-
tions. Your surgeon will probably tell you to avoid sex, heavy house-
work, alcohol, steam baths and saunas for at least two weeks, for
example. You'll also need to avoid the sun for several months.

Cosmetic Surgery Is Still Surgery

The idea of trading in your old face for a new one can be exhilarating. But don't forget: Cosmetic surgery is still surgery. And your doctor will need to make sure you're in top shape before she agrees to perform the procedure. "It's dangerous to present cosmetic surgery as something akin to having your nails done," says Dr. Cramer. "Cosmetic surgery is serious business."

Certain health conditions, like severe diabetes or emphysema, may rule out cosmetic surgery altogether. A surgeon will also ask you what prescription drugs you're taking, if any, and health conditions that might cause problems during and after the surgery, like high blood pressure, blood-clotting problems or a tendency to form scars. A surgeon will also want to know if you smoke; some doctors won't perform cosmetic procedures on smokers because they bruise more easily than nonsmokers and risk other side effects from surgery that nonsmokers don't.

After a surgeon is finished interviewing *you*, ask her to explain the risks of the procedure you're interested in. Generally speaking, the potential for complications is slim. But here's what can go wrong.

Scarring. Surgeons generally place incisions in skin folds. "That way, if incisions don't heal perfectly, they don't show, or you can at least hide them with makeup," says Dr. Cramer. But the outcome of cosmetic surgery is never completely predictable. "Even the best surgeon can't guarantee that you won't end up with a scar," says Dr. Rosenblatt.

Bleeding. Bleeding under the skin in the area of the surgery (called a hematoma) occurs in about 5 percent of people, usually within the first two days after surgery. Small hematomas go away on their own. Larger hematomas will need to be drained or surgically removed. "If hematomas aren't drained early enough, the resulting pressure can cause the skin to shed," says Dr. Pearlman (see below).

Skin sloughs. A skin slough is a section of skin that dies, scabs over and falls away. "About 15 percent of people who undergo a face-lift will get a skin slough behind their ears," says Dr. Pearlman. Small skin sloughs generally heal with no problem, she says. But larger ones may cause scarring.

Smokers are most likely to develop skin sloughs: "Nicotine constricts the blood supply, which the skin needs to heal," says Dr. Cramer.

Nerve damage. The deeper the face-lift, the greater the risk of nerve damage, says Dr. Rosenblatt. If nerve damage occurs, the eyelids or the muscles around the eyebrows are most likely to become paralyzed, says Dr. Pearlman. Sometimes the paralysis is temporary. But in rare cases, this paralysis can be permanent.

Other risks of cosmetic surgery include infection or blindness. But doctors say these complications are very rare.

Note: Cosmetic surgeons use general anesthesia (which renders you completely unconscious) or local anesthesia (which numbs only the area to be treated) along with a sedative to make you feel drowsy. Most cosmetic surgeons prefer to use local anesthesia because it causes fewer complications than general anesthesia. So you may want to ask a surgeon about what type of anesthesia she would use.

Do You Really Need Surgery?

Unlike corrective surgery, no one *needs* cosmetic surgery. But if you're thinking seriously about undergoing a face-lift or other cosmetic procedure, you need to ask yourself why you want it, say experts. More important, they say, you have to answer yourself honestly.

"The goal of cosmetic surgery is to enhance a person's self-esteem," says Paula A. Moynahan, M.D., attending plastic and reconstructive surgeon at Lenox Hill Hospital, and St. Mary's Hospital and Waterbury Hospital in Waterbury, Connecticut. But no matter how artful the surgery, perkier eyelids or a trimmer jawline can't cure depression or return you to the carefree days of your youth.

While you may know that getting an eye tuck is no guarantee of living happily ever after, some people may not. So don't be surprised if, during a consultation (see "Shopping for a Surgeon? Give 'Em the Third Degree" on page 258) a surgeon asks you what you expect to gain from surgery, how you feel your life may change afterward, even how you feel about your life in general. She wants to make sure that you'll enter into surgery with reasonable expectations.

"If a woman comes into my office with a picture of a young Elizabeth Taylor and says, 'I want to look like this,' that's a red flag," says Dr. Moynahan. Nor will she perform cosmetic surgery on a person recently widowed or divorced: "Cosmetic surgery won't fill that emotional void," she says.

The bottom line: You need to undergo cosmetic surgery for *you.* "You have to go into cosmetic surgery with realistic expectations," says Dr. Cramer. "Otherwise, it's a setup for disaster. The most important question to ask yourself is, 'Why do I want to do this?' The right answer is, 'Because I want to feel better about myself.' "

CHAPTER FORTY-EIGHT

Dermabrasion

Buff Away the Years

You may not know it, but every time you scrub your face with a washcloth, you slough away dead skin cells that can dull your complexion. This buffing process, called exfoliation, can give your skin a somewhat fresher look. What exfoliation can't do, of course, is help eliminate lines or wrinkles. But a cosmetic surgeon's version of exfoliation—called dermabrasion—can. In dermabrasion, a doctor uses a high-speed, rotating brush or other tool to literally sand away the outer layers of the skin.

Dermabrasion may sound like a drastic way to achieve younger-looking skin, but this procedure can be a useful tool—in the right hands. And the results can be dramatic: Dermabrasion can improve the texture and tone of coarse, leathery skin, remove age spots, eradicate some lines and wrinkles and soften very deep expression lines.

But dermabrasion is also a serious procedure that may not be appropriate for everyone. For the facts about dermabrasion, read on.

What Dermabrasion Can Do

When performed correctly, dermabrasion can deliver a host of benefits that help make skin look younger and fresher. "Dermabrasion removes the weathered skin. The new skin that forms has a much more youthful appearance," says John M. Yarborough, M.D., clinical professor of dermatology at Tulane University School of Medicine in New Orleans.

This procedure may also help the skin generate collagen, the substance that helps keep skin firm and youthful-looking, says Dr. Yarborough. "Dermabrasion can eradicate much of the sun-damaged collagen and help new collagen to form."

Dermabrasion can also improve the appearance of scars, including scars that are a legacy of youthful bouts with acne. "You may need to undergo dermabrasion more than once if the scars are very deep," says Dr. Yarborough, but many patients are satisfied with the results of one treatment. While older scars are harder to eradicate completely, it's possible to completely remove new scars if they're treated within one to two months.

What to Expect

With over 15,000 dermabrasion procedures to his credit, Dr. Yarborough is acknowledged by cosmetic surgeons and dermatologists as one of the leading dermabrasion specialists in the country. Here's how he performs dermabrasion. Keep in mind, however, the doctors you consult may perform the procedure slightly differently.

To help people relax, Dr. Yarborough administers a sedative by injection. Some doctors may use intravenous anesthesia. Then he chills the skin with crushed ice or an ice pack to prepare it for a chemical spray that both anesthetizes and freezes the skin and creates a rock-hard surface to dermabrade. Some doctors don't use the spray and inject local anesthesia that blocks the nerves in the area of the dermabrasion for the length of the procedure. Others use both the spray and the injections.

Dr. Yarborough then dermabrades skin with a high-speed wire brush. Other doctors may use a tool called the diamond-studded fraise. Dr. Yarborough usually won't dermabrade the eyelids because the skin is so thin.

After the procedure, Dr. Yarborough covers the skin with Vigilon, a soothing dressing that looks much like plastic wrap. Vigilon reduces healing time and does away with the need for pain medicine after the procedure, says Dr. Yarborough. Patients come back the next day so he can change the dressing, and again in another two days.

The third day after dermabrasion, he tells people to apply petroleum jelly to the skin so it won't form a crust. Experts believe skin heals better if it doesn't scab over. After about a week, dermabraded skin looks like it has a sunburn. It takes three months for the skin to regain its normal color.

Dermabrasion or Peel? It Depends on Your Skin

Dermabrasion and the chemical peel are two of the most common procedures to help eradicate lines and wrinkles. But which best suits your skin? Here's what experts say.

If you have medium or dark skin . . . Opt for dermabrasion, advise most experts. "Deep peels can work well on fair skin," says John M. Yarborough, M.D., clinical professor of dermatology at Tulane University School of Medicine in New Orleans. "But peels can produce more severe pigment changes in medium- or dark-complexioned people than dermabrasion."

If you want to eliminate whistle lines . . . Most experts recommend dermabrasion for these tiny lines that form above the upper lip. "These lines are resistant even to deep peels," says Kevin S. Pinski, M.D., dermatologist, cosmetic surgeon and assistant professor at Northwestern University Medical Center in Chicago. "And to be effective with a peel, you run the risk of scarring."

If you're African American . . . Harold E. Pierce, Jr., M.D., dermatologist and cosmetic surgeon at the Pierce Cosmetic Surgery Center in Philadelphia and professor emeritus of dermatologic cosmetic surgery at Howard University in Washington, D.C., recommends a medium-depth peel to eliminate wrinkles and sun damage. If you want to eliminate acne or other scars, Dr. Pierce recommends a medium peel, then dermabrasion.

See also the chapter on chemical peels (chapter 45).

Want Lasting Results? Change Your Evil Ways

If you want the effects of dermabrasion to last, you'll need to stop doing whatever led to wrinkles in the first place, like sunbathing, smoking or both. "If the bad habits don't change, the lines will come back," says Dr. Yarborough.

You must avoid the sun for at least three solid months after dermabrasion, says Dr. Yarborough. "That means no Caribbean vacations, no raking leaves, even on a cloudy day." Why? Because the cells that produce melanin (the stuff that gives skin its pigment) don't all rejuvenate at the same time, and dermabraded skin may develop pigment problems if exposed to the sun too soon. "If you get a slight burn, your skin can develop splotchy dark patches, called hyperpigmentation," explains Dr. Yarborough. "If you get a serious burn, skin can develop hypopigmentation—permanently light patches. It's foolish to go through dermabrasion if you're not going to protect your skin from the sun."

You'll also need to wear a sunscreen or sunblock with a sun protection factor (SPF) of at least 15 every time you venture outdoors, even if you're just driving from home to the office. Sunlight can penetrate your windshield. In windy weather, you'll need to protect your face with a scarf or a hooded coat or jacket.

If you exercise, resume workouts slowly, advises Dr. Yarborough. You can do a light workout, like riding a stationary bike at an easy tension, seven to ten days after dermabrasion, he says. But take it easy: "Strenuous activity—high-impact aerobics, lifting weights, anything that causes you to grunt and grimace—can burst fragile capillaries in the face," says Dr. Yarborough. Also, avoid lifting anything heavy: "Get someone else to carry a heavy basket of laundry upstairs," he suggests.

And if you smoke, stop. Nicotine constricts the blood vessels in the face, which starves the skin of oxygen. You already know what smoking does to your general health.

The Down Side of Dermabrasion

After dermabrasion, skin may erupt in milia. These little white bumps (possibly tiny particles of the epidermis, the outermost layer of skin) become embedded in the skin during dermabrasion. Milia are temporary, says Dr. Yarborough. "They often show up four to six weeks after the dermabrasion and may take three to four months to go away." Experts aren't sure why, but many people who resume their use of Retin-A (topical tretinoin), the prescription vitamin A cream used to treat wrinkles, a week or two after dermabrasion find that the drug helps keep milia from forming.

Also, some people's skin may develop hypopigmentation (light spots) or hyperpigmentation (dark spots). People with very white or black skin are less likely to experience pigment changes, says Dr. Yarborough. But people of Mediterranean, Latin or Asian ancestry or lighter-skinned African Americans often experience some degree of hyperpigmentation. Dermabrasion creates a surgical brush burn, an injury Dr. Yarborough speculates stimulates skin to form melanin much the way a sunburn can start the tanning process. Using a prescription-strength skin-bleaching cream can correct the hyper-pigmentation in three to five weeks.

A small percentage of people who undergo dermabrasion will be left with somewhat lighter skin, says Dr. Yarborough. "Short of using corrective makeup, we don't know how to darken skin."

Because of dermabrasion's potential to cause pigment changes, many experts suggest people undergo dermabrasion over the entire face rather than opting for a spot treatment, like above the upper lip, that may turn lighter or darker than the skin around it. "I encourage people with medium or darker skin tones to get a full-face derma-brasion," says Dr. Yarborough. "I dermabrade from the hairline down to about a finger's breadth below the jaw. If there's a line of de-marcation, you'd have to be almost lying down for anyone to see it."

It's ironic that a procedure that can eliminate scars can conceiv-ably cause them. But scarring is a possibility, although minor.

People who take the acne drug Accutane (isotretinoin) may be more likely to develop scars after dermabrasion, perhaps because Accutane affects the oil glands, which play a part in the healing process. While no one has proven that there's a connection between taking Accutane and postdermabrasion scarring, most doctors will not perform dermabrasion while you're taking this drug or for any-where from six months to two years after you've stopped.

CHAPTER FORTY-NINE

Laser Treatment

Zap the Signs of Aging

*I*n case it's been a few years since you've studied physics, *laser* stands for Light Amplification by Stimulated Emission of Radiation. The beam of light emitted by a supermarket price code scanner is one of the simplest forms of laser. But doctors are using laser beams to treat more and more conditions, like ulcers and cataracts, and to perform procedures like gallbladder surgery. What's more, lasers can correct surface flaws that contribute to a prematurely aged look, like age spots, broken capillaries and minor wrinkles. The beauty of it is, lasers can treat these imperfections without harming flawless skin. (Some cosmetic surgeons even use laser beams instead of scalpels to perform face-lifts and eye tucks.)

Laser surgeons say that laser beams can de-age the skin the way dermabrasion, chemical peels and traditional cosmetic surgery can—but without the swelling, bruising and extensive recovery time these procedures typically require. Further, lasers are virtually painless, says Gregory S. Keller, M.D., a facial, plastic and laser surgeon in private practice in Santa Barbara, California. "A laser pulse feels like the snap of a rubber band against your skin."

While lasers may seem like the next best thing to a magic wand, don't be misled: Despite what you may have heard elsewhere, lasers can't cure every skin woe. Nor is this procedure 100 percent risk-free.

But if you want to get rid of a troublesome skin flaw that makes you look—and feel—older than you'd like, you may want to consider laser surgery.

Ready, Aim, Fire!

Detailed explanations of exactly how lasers work are best left to medical textbooks. Basically, though, laser light changes into intense heat and fries the flaw, destroying it on contact.

Here's how doctors interviewed for this book are using laser beams to de-age the skin. Your doctor can tell you more.

Age Spots

Lasers of choice: High-energy pulsed CO_2 laser; copper vapor laser; Q-switched YAG laser; KTP laser.

How it works: Laser light eliminates pigmented cells while by-passing flawless skin.

Average number of treatments needed: One or two, depending on the number of spots and their degree of pigmentation.

Healing period: Most age spots peel away one to two weeks after the procedure.

How other treatments compare: "Freezing age spots with liquid nitrogen (cryotherapy) is more likely to cause hypopigmentation, or abnormally lightened skin, than lasers," says Laurence M. David, M.D., president of the International Society of Cosmetic Laser Surgeons and chief of laser surgery at the Institute of Cosmetic and Laser Surgery in Hermosa Beach, California.

Additional comments: Your doctor may have you pretreat age spots with one of several chemical acids for a month before laser treatment, give spots an in-office chemical peel immediately before the procedure, or both.

Face-Lift or Eye-Lift

Laser of choice: High-energy pulsed CO_2 laser.

How it works: The laser makes the incision and cuts away excess skin, muscle and fat.

Average number of treatments needed: Just one. It takes a laser surgeon about three hours to perform a face-lift and about an hour to do an eye-lift.

Healing period: Most people who opt for a laser face-lift or eye-lift can return to work a week after the procedure.

How other treatments compare: Cosmetic surgery performed with lasers causes less bruising than conventional cosmetic surgery, says Dr. Keller. "The laser seals the blood vessels, so bleeding is greatly reduced. Less bleeding means less bruising." Also, lasers seal the lymphatic channels—the skin's "drainage system"—so fluid doesn't leak into surrounding tissues, which reduces swelling, he says.

Additional comments: You may have to search a bit before you find a surgeon who performs face-lifts or eye-lifts with a laser (see below for more information on how to select a qualified laser surgeon).

Lines and Wrinkles

Laser of choice: High-energy pulsed CO_2 laser.

How it works: Laser light can soften the edges of a wrinkle and stimulate certain cells—called fibroblasts—to generate collagen, which fills in the wrinkle. (Collagen is the material that helps keep skin youthfully smooth and taut.) Lasers work particularly well on crow's-feet around the eyes and the vertical whistle lines above the upper lip, says Dr. Keller.

Average number of treatments needed: One or two. "Superficial lines usually disappear completely," says Dr. David.

Healing period: Usually one week. "After the procedure, your skin will look slightly sunburned," says Dr. David. "When your skin returns to its normal color, the lines are gone."

How other treatments compare: In Dr. Keller's view, lasers can eliminate whistle lines better than dermabrasion: "There's less chance of hypopigmentation." And unlike with a chemical peel, a doctor can regulate how deeply a laser beam penetrates the skin. "With a peel, a doctor doesn't have that degree of control," says Dr. David.

Additional comments: Lasers can also soften deep expression lines. But don't expect miracles: "Some wrinkles are so deep that there's no collagen left to stimulate," says Dr. David.

Port-Wine Stains

Laser of choice: Flash pump dye laser.

How it works: Caused by an overgrowth of enlarged blood vessels, a port-wine stain is a large reddish-purple birthmark, usually located on the face, head or neck. (Think of Mikhail Gorbachev's forehead.) Certain types of laser light can absorb the red pigment in blood and help destroy these vessels: "The darker a port-wine stain, the better it absorbs laser light," says Dr. David. Doctors also use lasers to remove enlarged blood vessels caused by rosacea (pronounced ro-ZAY-shuh), a skin condition sometimes mistaken for acne.

Averge number of treatments needed: Three to five. But the number of treatments needed depends on the size of the flaw, say experts.

Healing period: Most doctors schedule laser treatments one month apart so skin has time to heal.

How other treatments compare: In the past, doctors froze, scraped away (curettage) or even surgically removed port-wine stains—treatments that frequently replaced pigmented skin with a scar. But newer lasers can eliminate these pigmented patches with little or no scarring.

Additional comments: While laser treatment can't always completely remove port-wine stains, says Dr. Keller, "the laser can usually reduce a port-wine stain to the point where you can cover it with normal makeup instead of a heavy camouflage makeup," he says.

Scars

Laser of choice: High-energy pulsed CO_2 laser.

How it works: Lasers fill in "ice pick" scars by triggering the production of collagen, as well as flattening and de-coloring raised, red or brown scars. Lasers can also abrade the edges of shallow acne scars, which softens their appearance.

Average number of treatments needed: Usually one.

Healing period: Ice pick scars generally heal in a week. Raised scars heal in one to two weeks.

How other treatments compare: The laser tends to improve the appearance of a scar better than dermabrasion or a chemical peel, says Dr. David.

Additional comments: Shallow acne scars don't heal as quickly as other types of scars. "It may take a year for these scars to show maximum improvement," says Dr. David.

Spider Veins

Laser of choice: Copper vapor laser; argon laser; KTP laser.

How it works: Laser light vaporizes these small but unsightly veins, which are often found on or around the nose or cheeks.

Average number of treatments needed: Usually one.

Healing period: Usually none. But skin will take a few more days to heal if the treated area develops a scab, says Dr. David.

How other treatments compare: Spider veins zapped with a laser don't scar as much as those treated with electrodesiccation, in which a doctor "electrocutes" errant veins with an electric needle. "A laser targets these veins more accurately," says Dr. David.

Additional comments: The Food and Drug Administration is reviewing a new laserlike technology called Photoderm, which in clinical tests eradicated varicose veins less than the thickness of a pencil. The manufacturers of Photoderm claim that recovery from this procedure is quicker than from sclerotherapy, in which a doctor destroys leg veins by injecting them with a solution. Photoderm may also eliminate browning and matting—temporary but unsightly skin reactions that sometimes occur at the site of the injection.

Know the Risks—And Your Doctor

Laser surgery's potential risks include temporary discoloration of the treated area, permanent darkening or lightening of the skin, scarring and infection. You should also know that about 5 percent of people who undergo laser therapy to remove a port-wine stain develop a scar. So weigh this procedure's perceived benefits against its potential risks.

Should you decide to undergo a laser procedure, choose a doctor carefully: At this writing, there's no national licensing or certification for laser surgery, so doctors can buy and use any laser regardless of whether they've been trained to use it. Here's how the experts suggest you proceed.

Schedule a consultation. Interview a prospective surgeon. Check her qualifications. Ask questions about the treatment you're interested in. "Ask a surgeon what kind of laser procedures she performs and how regularly," recommends Dr. David.

Review a surgeon's résumé. During the consultation, ask for a copy of the surgeon's résumé, called a curriculum vitae. "Check for training that relates to the laser, like a preceptorship—a course that has doctors work alongside a skilled laser specialist for a certain amount of time," advises Dr. David.

The more lasers, the better. "Surgeons who have more than one laser system or who work at a laser center generally have a good amount of laser experience," says Dr. Keller. Similarly, you may want to avoid surgeons who use one laser to treat every skin flaw.

See also the chapters on age spots and freckles (chapter 1), chemical peels (chapter 45), cosmetic surgery (chapter 47) and dermabrasion (chapter 48).

CHAPTER FIFTY

Liposuction

More than Just a "Thigh Helper"

$\mathcal{M}$ention liposuction and most people automatically think of saddlebag thighs sucked clean of every morsel of excess fat. And liposuction can and is used to slim down thighs. But resourceful doctors have also found liposuction to be a handy way to defat wiggly areas elsewhere—annoying features like a double chin, jowls or other pouches of fat that you *know* you didn't have back when you were studying logarithms in 11th grade.

Besides trimming a double chin, puffy neck or jowls, liposuction—in which a surgeon uses a thin, hollow metal tube called a cannula to aspirate, or suck away, body fat through small incisions in the skin—can also streamline problem areas like the hips, stomach and buttocks and improve the appearance of cellulite, that rippled, orange-peel-textured fat. And unlike dieting, which merely reduces the size of fat cells, liposuction gets rid of these cells permanently.

Like any other type of cosmetic surgery, liposuction entails some risk. But experts say a technique developed within the past few years has significantly reduced this procedure's potential for complications. So if you want a trimmer jawline, chin or neck or a sleeker figure, liposuction might be right for you.

Great Aspirations

Liposuction (doctors call it suction-assisted lipectomy) originated in Italy in the mid-1970s and emigrated to the United States in the early 1980s. But back then, liposuction was risky: People chanced trading excess fat for permanently dimpled skin that looked (ironically) like cellulite. Further, traditional liposuction depended on general anesthesia—the kind that acts on the brain and central nervous system, rendering you completely unconscious. (General anesthesia tends to cause more complications than local anesthesia, which numbs only the area to be treated.) Worst of all, liposuction often caused severe blood loss, and people who underwent this procedure often needed blood transfusions.

Within the past few years, however, most surgeons have stopped administering traditional liposuction and use a newer procedure called tumescent liposuction. In this procedure, a surgeon injects the area with a special solution to make fatty tissue "tumesce," or swell up. This solution contains a local anesthetic to numb the area being treated, a chemical that temporarily shrinks capillaries to minimize blood loss and a drug that lessens bruising and swelling.

Performed correctly, tumescent liposuction is virtually painless, says Jeffrey A. Klein, M.D., assistant clinical professor of dermatologic surgery at the University of California at Irvine and a cosmetic surgeon in San Juan Capistrano, California, who developed the procedure. What's more, you'll be able to leave the doctor's office a half-hour after the procedure. (Some people can even drive themselves home, says Dr. Klein.) You'll feel sore 10 to 16 hours after the procedure as the anesthesia wears off. But you can usually ease this discomfort with an over-the-counter pain reliever. You'll also have to wear two elastic support garments for two to five days until your skin contracts along your new, trimmer contours.

The most important benefit of tumescent liposuction is safety: This procedure significantly reduces blood loss to a few tablespoons and completely eliminates the complications that can arise from general anesthesia. Many experts agree: "Tumescent liposuction is safer and more predictable than traditional liposuction," says Dwight Scarborough, M.D., assistant clinical professor at Ohio State University and a dermatologic surgeon in Dublin, Ohio.

Like any medical procedure, tumescent liposuction does have certain risks (see below). But tumescent liposuction also tends to produce better results than the older procedure. Dr. Klein's procedure causes less bruising and swelling than traditional liposuction, says Kevin S. Pinski, M.D., dermatologist, cosmetic surgeon and assistant professor at Northwestern University Medical Center in Chicago: Less trauma to the skin means you'll heal faster. What's more, doctors can use smaller cannulas than in traditional liposuction. The smaller tools remove fat more precisely, reducing the risk of permanently dimpled skin.

Using smaller cannulas also leaves intact the fibrous attachments that anchor skin to underlying tissues. "During the healing process, these fibrous tissues pull skin back to where it's supposed to go," says Dr. Klein. "I've had patients who were playing tennis within a week after the procedure." The bigger cannulas used in traditional liposuction often broke these fibrous attachments, says Dr. Klein—the reason why people had to wear a support garment for six weeks.

Perk Up Your Profile

If you want to trim down a double chin, puffy neck or jowls, facial liposuction could be an option. In this procedure, a surgeon suctions away excess fat in the chin and neck, and skin redrapes itself as it heals. This procedure, which uses local anesthesia, takes less than an hour, and you may see its slimming effects almost as quickly. "You can go back to normal activities the next day, minus your jowls," says Dr. Klein.

Facial liposuction works best for people in their thirties or forties whose skin is still tight and resilient enough to snap back on its own, says James W. Smith, M.D., professor of plastic and reconstructive surgery at New York Hospital–Cornell Medical Center in New York City. But if your facial skin is slightly lax, a surgeon may suggest a minilift. Developed by Dr. Scarborough and Emil Bisaccia, M.D., associate professor of medicine and dermatology at Columbia University in New York City, the minilift eliminates a double chin, jowls *and* loose skin. (A surgeon will first evaluate your skin and bone structure to see if you're a good candidate for this procedure.)

In a minilift, a surgeon suctions away excess fat in the chin and neck. Then she makes incisions in front of each earlobe, removes the fat pads in the jowls, extends the incisions to the back of the ears and stitches sagging tissues into place. After the surgery, your face will be bruised and swollen, and you'll have to wear a facial support garment (which looks much like a sling) for a week to ten days. Stitches come out in about five days. "After the tenth day, with a little makeup, you're ready to face the world," says Dr. Bisaccia.

As the swelling subsides, your new, trimmer chin and jawline will begin to emerge. "You'll see 80 percent of what you'll ultimately look like three months after the procedure and be completely healed in six months," says Dr. Bisaccia.

Good-bye Saddlebags and Love Handles

Liposuction can do more than pare down a puffy profile. This procedure can also eliminate stubborn fat on the hips, thighs, stomach, upper arms, calves, knees and ankles. Liposuction can also slim hips and thighs by one or two sizes. (Good news if your bottom half has always been a size or two larger than your top half, making it hard to find a suit or dress that fits.)

What's more, it's possible to see the benefits of this procedure immediately, says Dr. Klein: "You can look thinner the next day." You'll see 95 percent of what you'll ultimately look like in four to six weeks, as swelling fades and incisions heal, adds Dr. Klein.

Liposuction isn't the lazy woman's way to an svelte figure, though: There's still no substitute for a prudent diet and regular exercise. "Liposuction is not a treatment for general obesity," says Dr. Klein. And while smaller cannulas can help minimize the look of cellulite, tumescent liposuction can't work miracles: "Liposuction won't eliminate cellulite, but it can improve its appearance," says Dr. Klein.

Know the Risks

Experts say that tumescent liposuction has significantly reduced the two biggest risks of traditional liposuction—blood loss and complications arising from the use of general anesthesia. But they add that tumescent liposuction, like any type of surgery, carries inherent risks, including dimpled skin, permanent numbness in the treated area, scarring and an allergic reaction to the local anesthesia. So talk to a surgeon about this procedure's potential for complications during your initial consultation.

As for traditional liposuction, most surgeons no longer perform this procedure. But in addition to the risks mentioned above, you should know that it can also result in permanent darkening of the skin (hyperpigmentation), nerve damage, infection and shock (depending on the amount of fat removed).

Getting Full-Service Liposuction

Many surgeons say they perform tumescent liposuction. But not all doctors administer the procedure from beginning to end. Why? Because tumescent liposuction can take up to 5 hours to perform, depending on how much fat is removed. (Just injecting the solution can take 2½ hours.) "Following this procedure to the letter takes longer, and some doctors may not want to take the time," says Dr. Klein.

Here's what to ask your doctor during your consultation.

What size cannulas will you use? Traditional cannulas are only the diameter of your little finger. But Dr. Klein uses cannulas less than ⅛ inch in diameter to suction body fat and even smaller cannulas to perform facial liposuction. It's especially important that a surgeon use the smallest cannulas possible if you're looking to improve the appearance of cellulite, says Dr. Klein.

Will I need to donate blood in advance? If the surgeon says yes, chances are she isn't using the tumescent technique and your donation is in anticipation of a blood transfusion, says Dr. Klein.

Will you use general or local anesthesia? In addition to the local anesthetic in the tumescent solution, some doctors offer intravenous (IV) sedation, which allows people to sleep through the procedure.

While IV sedation is still considered local anesthesia, Dr. Klein prefers that it not be used. And if a surgeon uses general anesthesia, beware, says Dr. Klein: "General anesthesia carries the most risks, and using it is a fairly good indication that you won't get the true tumescent technique," he says.

Needless to say, despite the relative safety and benefits of tumescent liposuction, it's an elective procedure, and the cardinal rules apply: Think carefully about *all* the pros and cons; weigh the very real risks against the expected benefits; and be sure this procedure is right for you, given your individual health and financial condition.

CHAPTER FIFTY-ONE

Retin-A

The "Wonder Drug" for Wrinkles

When a new acne medication, Retin-A (topical tretinoin), was introduced in 1969, people doing battle with adult acne applauded. But when a medical journal reported that this simple cream also got rid of wrinkles, phones started ringing off the hook in dermatologists' offices everywhere . . . and never stopped.

Compared to many over-the-counter wrinkle creams that promised—and failed—to eliminate wrinkles, Retin-A sounded like a true wonder drug. And that's the catch: It works, but it is a drug. What's more, despite the fact that dermatologists have prescribed Retin-A to treat wrinkles for years, this drug is still officially approved as an acne medication only.

Most important, Retin-A is only effective if you protect your skin in other ways. Here's how Retin-A works.

The Terminator of Wrinkle Creams

As an acne treatment, Retin-A, a synthetic derivative of vitamin A, breaks down the intercellular glue that holds clumped cells together and helps expel the blackheads and whiteheads from which pimples develop. But when the creator of Retin-A, Albert M. Kligman, M.D., Ph.D., and his colleagues at the University of Pennsylvania School of Medicine began to study Retin-A's seeming power to rejuvenate skin, they—and subsequent researchers—found that Retin-A provided a host of skin-renewing benefits.

Retin-A stimulates the production of collagen, the sturdy substance that gives skin its taut, youthful look. Further studies suggested that Retin-A can increase the number of collagen ropes that anchor the skin's outer layer, the epidermis, to its inner layer, the dermis. The more of these ropes skin possesses, the less wrinkled it appears. Retin-A encourages the growth of new blood vessels, which makes skin look pinker and healthier, and sloughs away dead skin cells, exposing fresh, new skin underneath. Retin-A can also lighten age spots or eradicate them altogether. What's more, Retin-A can help eliminate growths called actinic keratoses, which are caused by sun damage, even before you can see them.

How Retin-A Works

Retin-A comes in gel, liquid or cream. For wrinkle reduction, most dermatologists prescribe the cream. It is also formulated in various strengths; your doctor will determine which is best for you.

Using Retin-A is a snap: You simply apply it to clean, bare skin at bedtime. Retin-A doesn't replace your regular moisturizer, however. "Retin-A becomes part of your total skin-care routine," says Dr. Kligman. After six months or so, your dermatologist will most likely tell you to use Retin-A on the weekends only. It generally takes six to ten months—maybe longer—to see maximum results. But you will see visible improvement during this time: "The more damaged your skin, the more improvement you'll see," says Dr. Kligman.

Some dermatologists have people use the highest concentration of Retin-A their skin can tolerate, because the stronger the formula, the faster the results. On the other hand, the more potent the formula, the more noticeable the side effects: red, irritated, scaly skin. (Renova—a formulation of Retin-A in a moisturizing cream base that helps to prevent irritation—is now awaiting approval from the Food and Drug Administration.) Other doctors start people on a lower dose of Retin-A to avoid these possible side effects. "My patients don't usually have any problem with Retin-A," says Melvin L. Elson, M.D., medical director of the Dermatology Center in Nashville and co-author of *The Good Look Book*.

Your skin should adjust to Retin-A within a month. You can help hide redness and scaliness with makeup, says Dr. Elson. "But if skin is broken, you need to see your dermatologist," he says. And if your skin is really uncomfortable, your doctor may have you cut back applications to every other night.

Retin-A also makes skin exquisitely sensitive to the sun. So it's important to apply a sunscreen or sunblock with a sun protection factor (SPF) of at least 15 every day (see below).

Not Just for Wrinkles Anymore

Besides helping to improve the effects of sun damage, Retin-A works in tandem with other cosmetic treatments. Dermatologists

What's in a Name?

In the skin-care section of your drugstore, you see a moisturizer that says it's formulated with vitamin A. Does that mean it's just as effective as Retin-A?

No. But to understand why requires a mini-lesson in chemistry. In a nutshell, the term *retinoids* refers to all drugs made with vitamin A (retinol). Retin-A is vitamin A that's been converted into an acid. By contrast, most over-the-counter creams and moisturizers are formulated with pure vitamin A or retinyl compounds like retinyl palmitate or retinyl acetate, yet another form of vitamin A—neither of which works like Retin-A, says Melvin L. Elson, M.D., medical director of the Dermatology Center in Nashville and co-author of *The Good Look Book*.

"Vitamin A is a very unstable molecule and may lose its value when combined with other ingredients," says Dr. Elson. "There's no over-the-counter product that contains the right vitamin A molecule that helps protect against photoaging. These drugstore products are vitamin A creams with no data to confirm their claims."

Since Retin-A generally costs the same or less than exclusive department store skin creams, adds Dr. Elson, there's no reason not to try the one product proven to help fight the effects of photoaging.

and cosmetic surgeons also have people pretreat their skin with Retin-A two weeks to a month before they undergo certain cosmetic procedures. "When skin is treated with Retin-A before the heavier facial peels, it rejuvenates more quickly," says Steven J. Pearlman, M.D., facial plastic surgeon and president of the New York Facial Plastic Surgery Society in New York City.

Retin-A also helps improve skin flaws unrelated to sun damage. Used quickly enough, this drug can help fade stretch marks, especially those acquired during pregnancy. "There's no question that shortly after childbirth, when stretch marks are still shallow and red, you can improve them quite a bit," says Dr. Kligman.

You Still Have to Shun the Sun

While Retin-A can improve the appearance of photodamaged skin, if not actually repair the damage itself, it's only one tool that can help in your quest for younger-looking skin. To maximize the effects of Retin-A and to protect your skin, you need to use SPF 15 sunscreen every time you venture outdoors. An easy way to get your daily dose of sunscreen is to use a moisturizer with added SPF 15 sunscreen. Also, stay out of the sun between the hours of 10:00 A.M. and 3:00 P.M. if possible and wear protective clothing, including hats and sunglasses, whenever you're out in direct sun.

Also, make sure you have realistic expectations: Retin-A can't remove wrinkles the way an eraser rubs out pencil marks. Nor can it firm up sagging skin. "Retin-A is not a substitute for cosmetic surgery, which is necessary to resurface, reshape and redrape severely sun-damaged skin," says Dr. Kligman. "A doctor will evaluate your skin and give you some idea of whether Retin-A can help your wrinkles and to what degree."

If you stop using Retin-A, wrinkles may come back after about a year. But doctors say there seems to be no reason not to use Retin-A indefinitely. "As far as we know, there are no long-term side effects," says Dr. Elson. But because Retin-A is a relatively new drug, studies are inconclusive.

See also the chapters on cellulite (chapter 7), stretch marks (chapter 16), moisturizers (chapter 27), chemical peels (chapter 45) and dermabrasion (chapter 48).

Index

Note: **Boldface** references indicate boxed text.